RHEUMATISM AND MUSCULOSKELETAL DISORDERS



# RHEUMATOID ARTHRITIS

# RISK FACTORS, HEALTH EFFECTS AND TREATMENT OPTIONS

AMANDA MELLE
EDITOR

nova
Medical & Health

## NOTICE TO THE READER



**Library of Congress Cataloging-in-Publication Data**

ISBN: 978-1-53613-668-5

*Published by Nova Science Publishers, Inc. † New York*

# CONTENTS

# PREFACE

In *Rheumatoid Arthritis: Risk Factors, Health Effects and Treatment Options*, the authors open by discussing discuss which bDMARDS and tsDMARDS might be preferred in particular situations, for example in the setting of previous malignancy or in those with an increased risk of infection. Emphasis will be placed on practical solutions for the busy clinician. Following this, they discuss the prevalence and implications of co-morbid depression in RA patients and sub-groups, focusing on ethnic minorities. The barriers to identification of depression and the reasons for low utilization of mental health care resources among specific ethnic groups are analyzed, taking into account patient perceptions of depression and its association with RA. Lastly, the current knowledge about the contribution of smoking as a risk factor for RA development and the possible mechanism of action is reviewed. In addition, the authors highlight the association of smoking habits with clinical, serological, radiographic damage statuses and comorbidities of RA. The benefits of designed smoking cessation intervention on RA outcomes will also be discussed.

Chapter 1 - There is an increasing range of disease modifying anti-rheumatic drugs (DMARDS) available for the treatment of rheumatoid arthritis (RA). The biological DMARDS (bDMARDS) include anti-cytokine antagonists, which target tumour necrosis factor (TNF), (e.g., etanercept, adalimumab and golimumab) and the interleukin (IL)-6 receptor (e.g., tocilizumab or sarilumab). Other bDMARDS target specific cell types implicated in disease pathogenesis, such as B-lymphocytes (e.g., rituximab) or T-lymphocytes (e.g., abatacept). The synthetic DMARDS are divided into two sub-classes – conventional (csDMARDS, e.g., methotrexate and sulfasalazine) and targeted (tsDMARDS) such as the new oral agents tofacitinib or baricitinib, which inhibit specific pro-inflammatory enzymes. More bDMARDS and tsDMARDS are being evaluated in clinical trial and will reach the clinic over the next few years.

While bDMARDS and tsDMARDS have revolutionalised the treatment of RA, it is difficult for the clinician to know which agent to choose in the individual patient with RA. This chapter will discuss which bDMARDS and tsDMARDS might be preferred in particular situations, for example in the setting of previous malignancy or in those with an increased risk of infection. Emphasis will be placed on practical solutions for the busy clinician.

A significant proportion of patients fail to respond to a particular bDMARD (primary failure) or lose response over time (secondary failure). One possible mechanism for secondary failure is the development of neutralising anti-drug antibodies (ADAb). The likelihood of development of ADAb differs between bDMARDS. The implications of this phenomenon and the effect of ADAb will be discussed as well as measures to combat this.

Chapter 2 - It is increasingly recognized that patients with rheumatoid arthritis (RA) suffer from high rates of depression, which often remains undiagnosed and untreated. In fact, depression was highlighted as the most common comorbidity in a large study on RA patients from 17 countries. Ethnic minority RA patients are even more likely to experience depression and less likely to seek mental health care than other individuals with RA. Due to its high prevalence and profound impact on functional disability and quality of life, prompt recognition and management of depression is urgently needed in patients with RA, in order to ensure the highest possible physical and mental health and well-being. Rheumatologists will inevitably face the challenge of addressing depression among their patients. In this chapter, the authors will discuss the prevalence and implications of co-morbid depression in RA patients and sub-groups, focusing on ethnic minorities. The authors will explore the barriers to identification of depression and the reasons for low utilization of mental health care resources among specific ethnic groups, taking into account patient perceptions of depression and its association with RA. While it is clear that new multidisciplinary clinical protocols should be developed to include depression screening and treatment as part of the rheumatology visit, specific intervention strategies and delivery thereof may differ for diverse ethnic minority groups. The authors will examine potential intervention approaches, the evidence regarding their effectiveness and cultural acceptability as well as potential for uptake among ethnically diverse patient groups. The authors will further make recommendations on gaps in education for RA patients with regard to depression. A comprehensive approach to the management of both physical and mental health needs of RA patients can aid in improving patient overall quality of life. Numerous potential strategies could be successfully implemented within the rheumatology clinic setting to better identify co-morbid depression among RA patients generally, and among ethnic minority patients more specifically. Such interventions could help mitigate disability, improve quality of life, patient function and overall satisfaction.

Chapter 3 - Rheumatoid arthritis (RA), an immune-mediated disease, is characterized by joint inflammation and systemic manifestations, which affects up to 1% of the adult population. RA is thought to arise due to the interacting effects of genetic and environmental factors, resulting in changes in immune system function. The genetics of RA are complex, however, carriage of the human leukocyte antigen (HLA)-DRB1 shared epitope (SE) is the most important genetic risk factor for RA, responsible for approximately 40% of genetic susceptibility to the disease. A number of environmental risk factors contribute to RA susceptibility, such as smoking, infections, and periodontitis. Cigarette smoke represents a mixture of toxic substances including nicotine, carbon monoxide, carcinogens, organic compounds and free radicals. Smoking is suggested to have a vital role in the pathogenesis of RA and it is known to modulate the immune system both humoral and cellular autoimmunity through numerous mechanisms. Smoking is a strong generator of anti-cyclic citrullinated peptide antibody (ACPA) and is known to associate with rheumatoid factor (RF). Evidence showed that smoking interacts with HLA-DRB1 and it is responsible for increasing the susceptibility to develop RA, mainly seropositive-RA. Epidemiologic researches have demonstrated that the smoking rate amongst RA patients is higher than in matched populations and it differs with gender. Smoking status and intensity (number of cigarettes/day) modulate both RA disease severity and outcome. For several years, the evidence was restricted to active smokers, however recent works showed that the risk of development of RA is found to be elevated in both former and passive smokers. Moreover, passive smokers reported high disease activity levels than never smokers in RA patients. In addition to the detrimental effects of tobacco on RA manifestations, heavy smoking is associated with serious comorbidities that required hospitalizations. Patients with RA who smoke, experience high cardiovascular events and respiratory tract infections and through these diseases, smoking is responsible for a higher mortality rate. Smoking cessation should not just be encouraged according to the general health recommendation but should be tailored for RA patient specifically. Evidence demonstrated the potential benefits of smoking cessation at any time after RA diagnosis. In this chapter the authors will review the current knowledge about the contribution of smoking as a risk factor for RA development and the possible mechanism of action. In addition, the authors will highlight the association of smoking habits with clinical, serological, radiographic damage statuses and comorbidities of RA. The benefits of designed smoking cessation intervention on RA outcomes will be discussed.

In: Rheumatoid Arthritis
Editor: Amanda Melle

ISBN: 978-1-53613-668-5


*Chapter 1*

# THE BIOLOGICAL THERAPY OF RHEUMATOID ARTHRITIS

***Peter K. K. Wong,[*] PhD***
Mid-North Coast Arthritis Clinic and Rural Clinical School,
University of New South Wales, Coffs Harbour,
New South Wales, Australia

## ABSTRACT

There is an increasing range of disease modifying anti-rheumatic drugs (DMARDS) available for the treatment of rheumatoid arthritis (RA). The biological DMARDS (bDMARDS) include anti-cytokine antagonists, which target tumour necrosis factor (TNF), (e.g., etanercept, adalimumab and golimumab) and the interleukin (IL)-6 receptor (e.g., tocilizumab or sarilumab). Other bDMARDS target specific cell types implicated in disease pathogenesis, such as B-lymphocytes (e.g., rituximab) or T-lymphocytes (e.g., abatacept). The synthetic DMARDS are divided into two sub-classes – conventional (csDMARDS, e.g., methotrexate and sulfasalazine) and targeted (tsDMARDS) such as the new oral agents tofacitinib or baricitinib, which inhibit specific pro-

[*] Corresponding Author Email: pkkw12@gmail.com.

inflammatory enzymes. More bDMARDS and tsDMARDS are being evaluated in clinical trial and will reach the clinic over the next few years.

While bDMARDS and tsDMARDS have revolutionalised the treatment of RA, it is difficult for the clinician to know which agent to choose in the individual patient with RA. This chapter will discuss which bDMARDS and tsDMARDS might be preferred in particular situations, for example in the setting of previous malignancy or in those with an increased risk of infection. Emphasis will be placed on practical solutions for the busy clinician.

A significant proportion of patients fail to respond to a particular bDMARD (primary failure) or lose response over time (secondary failure). One possible mechanism for secondary failure is the development of neutralising anti-drug antibodies (ADAb). The likelihood of development of ADAb differs between bDMARDS. The implications of this phenomenon and the effect of ADAb will be discussed as well as measures to combat this.

## INTRODUCTION

Pharmacologic treatment of rheumatoid arthritis (RA) has been revolutionised by an increasing range of biologic disease modifying anti-rheumatic drugs (bDMARDS) and targeted synthetic (ts)-DMARDS (Table 1). The anti-cytokine antagonists targeting tumour necrosis factor (TNF)/TNF inhibitors (TNFi) were the first bDMARD class available and comprise etanercept (ETN), adalimumab (ADL), certolizumab pegol (CZP), infliximab (IFX) and golimumab (GOL). This family of targeted therapies was soon followed by the interleukin (IL)-6 receptor inhibitor tocilizumab (TCZ). Other bDMARDS target specific cell types implicated in disease pathogenesis, such as B-lymphocytes (rituximab, RTX) or T-lymphocytes (abatacept, ABA). Targeted synthetic DMARDS (tsDMARDS) such as the oral agent tofacitinib (TFN) and the newer baricitinib inhibit the Janus kinases, an enzyme family implicated in the inflammatory cascade.

Conventional synthetic DMARDS (csDMARDS) such as methotrexate (MTX), leflunomide (LFN), salazopyrine (SSZ), hydroxycholorquine (HCQ) and azathioprine (AZA) have been used for many years in the treatment of RA. While MTX still forms the “anchor drug,” both bDMARDS and tsDMARDS are now an essential component of best-practice treatment for RA [1, 2]. However, this is a rapidly changing field as newer bDMARDS, tsDMARDS and biosimilar DMARDS are continually being approved [3]. Each of the bDMARDS have similar response rates which decrease with increasing drug experience and mostly appear to have increased efficacy in combination with csDMARDS [2]. Despite their efficacy, bDMARD therapy is expensive [4]. This is concerning as the cost of healthcare in most developed countries is rapidly rising due to the ageing population and availability of more expensive pharmacologic therapies for a range of chronic diseases. In response, many national regulatory agencies have turned to cheaper biosimilar bDMARDS.

**Table 1. Targeted synthetic and biologic disease modifying anti-rheumatic drugs (DMARDS) currently available for the treatment of rheumatoid arthritis**

| | Mechanism of action | Agent |
|---|---|---|
| **Biologic DMARDS** | Tumour necrosis factor inhibition | Etanercept [ETN] |
| | | Adalimumab [ADL]<br>Infliximab [IFX]<br>Certolizumab pegol [CZP]<br>Golimumab [GOL] |
| | Interleukin-6 receptor inhibition | Tocilizumab [TCZ] |
| | T-cell co-stimulation blockade | Abatacept [ABA] |
| | B-cell depletion | Rituximab [RTX] |
| **Targeted synthetic DMARDS** | Janus kinase inhibitor | Tofacitinib [TFN] |
| | | Baricitinib |

## Limitations of Clinical Trials

For brevity, while this chapter will discuss only the key clinical trials for each bDMARD or tsDMARD, it is important to consider the limitations of clinical trials. Clinical trials enrol mostly Caucasian patients. Only a few trials have enrolled significant numbers of Asian patients, for example TOWARD (9-10% Asians) for TCZ [5] or PLANETRA (11.3-12.2% Asians) for CT-P13, an IFX biosimilar [6].

Most studies have enrolled patients with established RA which has been present for some years, for example 6.1-6.2 years in RAPID1 [7], 10.6-13 years in ARRIVE [8] and 7.7-8.6 years in ORAL SOLO [9]. Only a few trials have examined bDMARD use in patients with early RA, for example, CZP in C-EARLY (9.6-12.4 months since symptom onset) [10], ADL in PREMIER (0.7-0.8 years of RA) [11], ADL in OPTIMA (4-5 months of RA duration) [12] and ABA in AMPLE (RA duration 1.7-1.9 years) [13].

Patients enrolled in clinical trials often differ to those in everyday clinical practice. For example, the mean baseline body weight of patients receiving TCZ in SUMMACTA was 73-74 kg [14] and 72.1-74.1 kg and 67.9-68.9 kg, respectively, in those receiving ABA in the AVERT [15] and ALLOW [16] trials. These relatively low body weights may not be representative of patients seen in routine clinical practice – particularly in North America and Australia. This may be one explanation for the lack of efficacy of these drugs in some "real-life" patients.

Another limitation is that primary outcomes of most clinical trials are usually measured at six or 12 months despite RA being a chronic disease lasting many years [7-9, 15]. This means uncommon outcomes such as malignancy or death may not be adequately captured in a clinical trial. Long-term extension (LTE) studies seek to address this concern but usually suffer from "channelling bias" as they only include patients who respond and tolerate the drug of interest.

However, with these caveats in mind, randomised controlled clinical trials provide a powerful tool to evaluate the efficacy of novel therapeutic agents.

# ETANERCEPT

## Mechanism of Action

Etanercept was the first subcutaneously (SC) administered bDMARD for the treatment of RA. The molecule is a genetically engineered fusion protein comprising two identical chains of the recombinant human TNF-receptor p75 monomer fused with the fragment crystallisable (Fc) domain of human IgG1, which binds and inactivates TNF [17].

## Clinical Studies

### *Established RA (ETN + MTX)*

A double-blind study was undertaken to determine whether addition of ETN to MTX would provide additional benefit in patients with persistent RA (mean disease duration of 6·8 years) despite at least six months of MTX monotherapy [18]. Eighty-nine patients were randomised to receive either ETN 25 mg or placebo (PBO), given SC twice weekly while continuing MTX.

At 24 weeks, 71% of those receiving ETN + MTX and 27% of those receiving PBO + MTX had ACR20 (American College of Rheumatology [ACR] criteria 20% improvement) responses ($p < 0.001$) while 39% of those receiving ETN + MTX and 3% of those receiving PBO + MTX met ACR50 responses (ACR criteria 50% improvement) ($p < 0.001$) (Table 2). The only adverse events (AEs) significantly associated with ETN were mild injection site reactions (ETN + MTX 42% versus PBO + MTX 7%, $p < 0.001$). No patient withdrew from the study because of ETN associated AEs [18]. Non-neutralizing antibodies to ETN were detected in only one study patient.

The much larger TEMPO study randomized 686 patients with active RA to ETN 25 mg SC twice weekly (n = 212) or MTX < 20 mg/week (n = 212) or ETN + MTX (n = 218) [19]. At week 52, 85% (95% CI 80–89) of patients in the ETN + MTX group achieved ACR20 responses compared with 75% (95% CI 69–80) and 76% (95% CI 70–81) in the MTX and ETN groups, respectively ($p = 0{\cdot}01$ for ETN + MTX versus MTX alone; $p = 0{\cdot}015$ for ETN + MTX versus ETN alone) (Table 2) [19]. At week 52, 69% (95% CI 63–75) of those in the ETN + MTX group achieved ACR50 responses compared with 43% (95% CI 36–49) and 48% (95% CI 42–55) in the MTX and ETN monotherapy groups, respectively ($p < 0{\cdot}0001$ for ETN + MTX versus MTX alone; $p < 0{\cdot}0001$ for ETN + MTX versus ETN alone).

The mean change in Total Sharp Score (TSS) for the ETN + MTX group was lower than for the MTX and ETN monotherapy arms at week 52. The proportion of patients without radiographic progression at week 52 was higher in those receiving ETN + MTX compared to those who received ETN or MTX alone (80% [95% CI 74–85] versus 68% [95% CI 61–74] and 57% [95% CI 50–64], respectively; $p < 0{\cdot}0001$ for ETN + MTX compared to MTX alone and $p = 0{\cdot}004$ for ETN + MTX compared to ETN alone) [19].

***Early RA and Clinical Remission (ETN + MTX)***

The COMET study randomized 542 MTX-naive patients with early (symptoms present for 3–24 months, mean of nine months) moderate-to-severe RA to either MTX (≤ 20 mg/week) by week 8 or MTX + ETN 50 mg SC weekly [20].

At week 52, 132/265 (50%, 95%CI 44–56%) of those treated with ETN + MTX achieved clinical remission (disease activity score 28-joint count [DAS-28] < 2.6) compared to 73/263 (28%, 95%CI 23–33%) of those taking MTX alone (Table 2). One hundred and ninety six of 246 patients (80%, 95%CI 75–85%) and 135/230 (59%, 95%CI 53–65%), respectively achieved radiographic non-progression. The incidence of serious AEs was similar between the two groups. Importantly, those who received ETN + MTX had a nearly three-fold reduction in work stoppage due to RA compared with those on MTX alone [20].

At two-year follow-up, early sustained ETN + MTX therapy remained superior to MTX monotherapy for both clinical remission (DAS-28 < 2.6) and radiographic progression (modified Sharp/van der Heijde score (mTSS) [21]. There were no additional safety signals at two years.

### *Use of ETN + SSZ*

Most bDMARD trials have studied MTX as the primary csDMARD. However, SSZ is also widely used in clinical practice. Patients with active RA despite SSZ were randomised to ETN 25 mg twice weekly (n = 103), ETN + SSZ (n = 101, 2–3 g/day) or SSZ alone (n = 50) in a double-blind, randomised, two-year study [22]. At week 24, the ACR20 response was achieved by 74%, 74% and 28% of patients, respectively ($p < 0.01$) (Table 2). Benefit was seen from week 2 in those receiving ETN. The incidence of infection and injection site reactions was higher with ETN ($p < 0.05$) [22]. There was no therapeutic advantage to continuing SSZ following addition of ETN.

### *Withdrawal of ETN (PRESERVE)*

The above studies examined addition of ETN to csDMARDS in patients with incompletely controlled RA. The aim of the PRESERVE study was to determine whether the response to ETN + MTX could be sustained when ETN was dose reduced or withdrawn [23]. In an open-label "run-in" period of 36 weeks, all patients received ETN 50 mg/week + MTX. Those patients who achieved sustained low disease activity (LDA) were then randomized for a double-blind period of 52 weeks to one of three treatment groups: ETN 50 mg weekly + MTX, ETN 25 mg weekly + MTX or PBO + MTX. At Week 88, 166/201 (82·6%) patients who had received at least one dose of ETN 50 mg weekly and 159/201 (79·1%) patients given ETN 25 mg weekly had LDA, compared with 84/197 (42·6%) who had received PBO [23]. This complex but novel study showed that even sustained LDA required continuation of ETN – although a lower ETN dose appeared sufficient. As patients in PERSERVE had moderately active RA, results might not be generalizable to patients with early or severe disease.

**Table 2. Key clinical trials involving etanercept**

| Study | Time of primary efficacy end-point | Responses | Proportion (%) of patients in each group for each response measure | | | | | |
|---|---|---|---|---|---|---|---|---|
| | | | PBO + MTX | MTX alone | SSZ alone | ETN alone | ETN + MTX | ETN + SSZ |
| Weinblatt, 1999 [18] | Week 24<br>Week 24 | ACR20<br>ACR50 | 27<br>3 | | | | 71<br>39 | |
| TEMPO [19] | Week 52<br>Week 52 | ACR20<br>ACR50 | | 75<br>43 | | 76<br>48 | 85<br>69 | |
| COMET [20] | Week 52 | DAS-28 remission (< 2.6) | 28 | | | | 50 | |
| Combe, 2009 [22] | Week 24<br>Week 24 | ACR20<br>ACR50 | | | 28<br>14 | 77<br>47 | | 77<br>52 |

ACR20 = American College of Rheumatology criteria 20% improvement, ACR50 = American College of Rheumatology criteria 50% improvement, DAS-28 = Disease activity score 28-joint count, ETN = etanercept, PBO = placebo, MTX = methotrexate, SSZ = salazopyrine.

## Summary

Etanercept is an effective TNFi in combination with MTX for treatment of RA and is effective at inducing clinical remission in early RA. There appeared no therapeutic advantage to continuing SSZ following addition of ETN [22]. Although combination ETN + MTX is effective at achieving sustained LDA, continuation of ETN is required to maintain disease control – although a lower ETN dose may be used [23]. There appears to be a lower risk of mycobacterial infection with ETN compared to other TNFi's [24, 25]. Unlike the TNFi monoclonal antibodies (mAbs, i.e., ADL, IFX or GOL), ETN is not effective in the treatment of inflammatory bowel disease [26].

# ADALIMUMAB

## Mechanism

This was the first human (100% human peptide sequences) TNFi mAb available for the treatment of RA. Adalimumab blocks the interaction of TNF with the p55 and p75 TNF cell surface receptors [27].

## Clinical Trials

### *In MTX Inadequate Responders and MTX-Naïve Patients*

In a multicenter, 52-week, double-blind, PBO-controlled study, 619 patients with active RA and an inadequate response to MTX were randomised to receive ADL 40 mg SC every fortnight (n = 207), ADL 20 mg SC every week (n = 212), or PBO (n = 200), all in combination with MTX [28]. At week 24, ACR20 responses were achieved by 63.3% and 60.8% of patients taking ADL 40 mg every fortnight + MTX and ADL 20 mg weekly + MTX, respectively, versus 29.5% of patients taking

PBO + MTX ($p < 0.001$ for each comparison) (Table 3). There was significantly less radiographic progression, as measured by the change in TSS, in those receiving ADL at either dose compared with those receiving PBO ($p < 0.001$ for each comparison). The rate of AEs (including injection site reactions) was comparable in the ADL and PBO groups, although more serious infections were observed in those receiving ADL (3.8%) compared to PBO (0.5%, $p < 0.02$) [28]. Treatment with ADL was associated with a higher rate of antinuclear antibodies (ANA) and anti-dsDNA antibodies, but no cases of lupus or lupus-like illness were observed during the study [28].

Of the 619 patients randomised in the above study, 457 entered the open-label extension with 202 completing 10 years of follow-up [29]. Interestingly, at year 10 of follow-up, patients initially randomized to ADL + MTX had significantly lower mean mTSS compared to those who initially received PBO + MTX. This suggested than even a one year delay in commencing ADL + MTX was associated with reduced efficacy, suggesting a "window of opportunity" to prevent irreversible joint damage in RA. No new safety signals were observed during 10 years of ADL treatment [29].

The PREMIER study was a 2-year, multicenter, double-blind, controlled study of 799 RA patients of less than three years duration (mean duration 0.7 years) randomised to ADL 40 mg SC every fortnight + MTX, ADL 40 mg SC every fortnight as monotherapy or weekly MTX monotherapy [11]. At week 52, more patients receiving ADL + MTX had an ACR50 response (62%) than patients who received MTX or ADL monotherapy (46% and 41%, respectively; both $p < 0.001$) (Table 3). Less radiographic progression ($p < 0.002$) was seen in those on ADL + MTX compared to either of the monotherapy arms [11]. The overall rate of infectious AEs was similar between the three treatment groups.

Two hundred and fifty of 497 patients (50.3%) completed the 10-year LTE. While no new safety signals were observed, patients initially randomised to ADL + MTX had better outcomes, particularly in prevention of radiographic progression compared to monotherapy with either ADL or MTX [30].

***Use in Early RA – "Window of Opportunity"***

The OPTIMA study was a complex trial designed to test different treatment strategies in RA [12]. The initial aim was to assess outcomes of patients with early RA who achieved stable LDA with MTX + ADL compared to those receiving MTX + PBO. The next part of the trial then sought to determine in patients who achieved stable LDA, whether those who received initial combination therapy with ADL + MTX had better clinical and radiographic outcomes than those who received MTX alone. Therapeutic outcomes were then assessed following ADL withdrawal in those who initially responded to ADL + MTX.

In Period 1, 1032 MTX-naïve patients with active RA and disease duration from diagnosis of less than one year (mean 4-4.5 months) were randomised to ADL + MTX or PBO + MTX [12]. Treatment modifications were then made based on achievement of LDA (defined as DAS-28 C-reactive protein [DAS-28-CRP] < 3.2) at weeks 22 and 26. At week 24, 44% (n = 207/466) of those receiving ADL + MTX versus 24% (n = 112/460) of those who received PBO + MTX achieved stable LDA ($p < 0.001$). Overall, ADL + MTX was superior to MTX alone at achieving better ACR responses and more clinical remissions (Table 3), greater mean reductions in DAS-28-CRP, less radiographic progression, and normal functional status at week 26 ($p < 0.001$ for all comparisons). The frequency of AEs was similar between groups, although more serious infections (2.5% versus 1.2%) and deaths (1.2% versus 0.2%) occurred in the ADL + MTX compared to the PBO + MTX group, respectively [12].

In Period 2, patients in the ADL + MTX group who completed Period 1 and achieved stable LDA (DAS-28-CRP < 3·2 at weeks 22 and 26) were randomised to ADL-continuation or ADL-withdrawal for another 52 weeks [31]. Those achieving stable LDA with initial MTX continued this. Inadequate responders were offered ADL + MTX.

**Table 3. Key clinical trials involving adalimumab**

| Study | Time of primary efficacy end-point | Responses | Proportion (%) of patients in each group for each response measure | | | | | |
|---|---|---|---|---|---|---|---|---|
| | | | PBO + MTX | MTX alone | ADL alone | ADL + MTX | ADL (40 mg q2w) + MTX | ADL (40 mg q1w) + MTX |
| Keystone, 2004 [28] | Week 24 | ACR20 | 29.5 | | | | 63.3 | 60.8 |
| | Week 24 | ACR50 | 9.5 | | | | 39.1 | 41 |
| PREMIER [11] | Week 52 | ACR20 | | 63 | 54 | 73 | | |
| | Week 52 | ACR50 | | 46 | 41 | 62 | | |
| OPTIMA, Period 1 [12] | Week 26 | ACR20 | 57 | | | 70 | | |
| | Week 26 | ACR50 | 34 | | | 52 | | |
| | Week 26 | DAS-28-CRP < 3.2 | 17 | | | 34 | | |

ACR20 = American College of Rheumatology criteria 20% improvement, ACR50 = American College of Rheumatology criteria 50% improvement, DAS-28-CRP = Disease activity score 28-joint count C-reactive protein, ADL = adalimumab, PBO = placebo, MTX = methotrexate, q1w = every week; q2w = every two weeks.

Of the 466 patients in the ADL + MTX group who completed Period 1, 207 achieved stable LDA, of whom 105 were re-randomised to ADL-continuation and 102 to ADL- withdrawal. Of the 460 patients in the PBO + MTX group who completed Period 1, 112 achieved stable LDA and continued MTX-monotherapy. Seventy-three of 105 (70%) patients in the ADL-continuation group and 61 of 112 (54%) patients in the MTX-monotherapy group achieved the primary end-point at week 78 (p = 0·023). Patients achieving the stable LDA target with ADL + MTX who withdrew ADL mostly maintained their good responses at week 78. There was no difference in the rate of AEs between groups [31].

The most novel finding of this study was that early treatment with ADL + MTX during a "window of opportunity" seemed to allow successful ADL withdrawal – so-called "induction-maintenance" therapy. However, given that RA is usually a chronic disease, longer patient follow-up is probably required.

## Summary

Adalimumab was the first fully human TNFi used in the treatment of RA. Its efficacy, tolerability and robust track record have made it the most commonly prescribed bDMARD for treatment of inflammatory arthritis. Early use of ADL + MTX for the treatment of RA was well-tolerated and may allow subsequent withdrawal of ADL with little loss of therapeutic response [31].

# INFLIXIMAB

## Mechanism of Action

Infliximab is a chimeric human-murine mAb given intravenously (IV) which neutralises the biological activity of TNF by binding with high affinity to the soluble and transmembrane forms of TNF as well as inhibiting binding of TNF to its receptors [32].

## Clinical Trials

### *Use in MTX Inadequate Responders (ATTRACT)*

This was a double-blind PBO-controlled trial which randomised 428 patients with active RA despite MTX for at least three months to PBO (n = 88) or one of four regimens of IV IFX at weeks 0, 2, and 6 then every 4 or 8 weeks on a background of MTX [33]. At week 30, ACR20 response rates were achieved in 53, 50, 58, and 52% of patients receiving IV IFX 3 mg/kg every 4 or 8 weeks or IV IFX 10 mg/kg every 4 or 8 weeks, respectively, compared with 20% of patients receiving PBO + MTX ($p < 0{\cdot}001$ for each of the four IFX groups versus PBO) (Table 4). Therapeutic response was rapid, with over half the responders achieving ACR20 response by week 2, and about 90% by week 6. There was no difference in serious AEs or serious infections in those receiving IFX or PBO [33].

At week 102 of IFX + MTX, clinically relevant improvements in physical function and quality of life, inhibition of radiographic joint damage and sustained improvement in RA disease activity continued, with no difference in serious AEs in those who received MTX only (33%) compared to IFX + MTX (29%) [34].

### *Use in Early RA (ASPIRE)*

One thousand and forty-nine RA patients with disease duration less than three years (mean 0.8-0.9 years) were randomised to MTX + PBO, MTX + IFX 3 mg/kg or MTX + IFX 6 mg/kg [35]. Infusions were given at week 0, 2, and 6 and every 8 weeks until week 46. Patients receiving MTX + IFX 3 mg/kg and MTX + IFX 6 mg/kg achieved higher ACR responses rates compared to those receiving MTX + PBO with no difference between the two doses of IFX (Table 4). Infliximab was associated with a higher incidence of serious infections, especially pneumonia (2-3% compared to 0% for PBO). As for all the TNFi's, IFX was associated with development of ANAs. Overall, 118/298 patients (39.6%) in the MTX + IFX 3 mg/kg, 106/309 patients (34.3%) in the MTX + IFX 6 mg/kg group, and 29/256 patients (11.3%) in the MTX + PBO arms developed ANAs during the study ($p < 0.001$ for both IFX groups compared to the MTX + PBO group [35]. Anti-drug antibodies (ADAb) to IFX were detected in 46/317 patients (14.5%) and 21/312 patients (6.7%) in the MTX + IFX 3 mg/kg and MTX + IFX 6 mg/kg groups, respectively.

***Use in a "Real-Life" Patient Cohort (START)***

Patients with active RA despite MTX were randomised to PBO (group 1, n = 363), IFX 3 mg/kg (group 2, n = 360), or IFX 10 mg/kg (group 3, n = 361) with infusions at week 0, 2, 6, and 14 [36]. Unlike ATTRACT [33], co-morbidities affecting organs (renal, hepatic, haematologic, gastrointestinal, endocrine, pulmonary) were not excluded – providing a study cohort more representative of routine clinical practice.

The risk of serious infections in patients receiving IFX 3 mg/kg + MTX was similar to those receiving MTX alone. However, the higher dose of IFX 10 mg/kg + MTX was associated with an increased risk of serious infections. There was no clinically significant difference in efficacy between the IFX 3 mg/kg and 10 mg/kg doses [36].

Another component of the START study was that from week 22, patients in group 2 were able to have the IFX dose increased in increments of 1.5 mg/kg at week 22, 30, 38 and 46 if they failed to achieve a 20% improvement from baseline in the combined tender joint count (TJC) and swollen joint count (SJC). About two-thirds of patients did not require any dose escalation and received IFX 3 mg/kg throughout the 12-month study. Forty-one of 53 primary non-responders (77%) responded to dose escalation while of the 47 secondary non-responders, 39 (83%) responded to dose escalation [36]. There was no difference in AEs, especially infections, between those who underwent dose escalation compared to those who did not.

**Table 4. Key clinical trials involving infliximab**

| Study | Time of primary efficacy end-point | Responses | Proportion (%) of patients in each group for each response measure | | | | |
|---|---|---|---|---|---|---|---|
| | | | PBO + MTX | IFX (3 mg/kg) q4w/q8w | IFX (10 mg/kg) q4w/q8w | IFX (3 mg/kg) + MTX | IFX (6 mg/kg) + MTX |
| ATTRACT [33] | Week 30 | ACR20 | 20 | 53/50 | 58/52 | | |
| | Week 30 | ACR50 | 5 | 29/27 | 26/31 | | |
| ASPIRE [35] | Week 54 | ACR20 | 53.6 | | | 62.4 | 66.2 |
| | Week 54 | ACR50 | 32.1 | | | 45.6 | 50.4 |

ACR20 = American College of Rheumatology criteria 20% improvement, ACR50 = American College of Rheumatology criteria 50% improvement, IFX = infliximab, PBO = placebo, MTX = methotrexate, q4w = every four weeks; q8w = every eight weeks.

## Summary

While IFX ushered in the era of targeted therapy and is generally an effective treatment for RA, the IV route of administration can be inconvenient; especially given that a wide range of SC bDMARDS and oral tsDMARDS is now available. In routine clinical practice, some clinicians find the 3 mg/kg dose not sufficiently effective for the treatment of RA – especially if given every eight weeks. However, this may be the only dose funded for the treatment of RA by local regulatory bodies, for example in Australia.

# CERTOLIZUMAB PEGOL

## Mechanism of Action

Certolizumab pegol (CZP) is a recombinant, humanised antibody Fab' fragment which neutralises membrane-associated and soluble human TNF, fused to a polyethylene glycol moiety to prolong the *in vivo* half-life. It lacks an Fc region, which is normally present in a complete antibody, and therefore does not fix complement or cause antibody-dependent cell-mediated cytotoxicity *in vitro* [37]. Certolizumab pegol also does not induce *in vitro* apoptosis in human peripheral blood-derived monocytes or lymphocytes, or neutrophil degranulation [37].

## Clinical Trials

### *Key Randomized Controlled Trials*

The efficacy and safety of CZP were assessed in four key randomised, PBO-controlled, double-blind studies (RAPID1 [7], RAPID2 [38], FAST4WARD [39] and another led by Choy [40]) in adult patients with moderate-to-severe active RA.

The RAPID1 [7] and RAPID2 [38] studies were the pivotal clinical trials, which enrolled patients who had received MTX for at least six months but had an incomplete response to MTX monotherapy. Patients were treated with a loading dose of CZP 400 mg at weeks 0, 2 and 4 or PBO followed by either 200 mg or 400 mg of CZP or PBO every other week, in combination with MTX for 52 weeks in RAPID1 and 24 weeks in RAPID2. Patients were evaluated for clinical disease activity and structural damage using the ACR20 response criteria at week 24 (RAPID1 and RAPID2) and mTSS at week 52 (RAPID1).

In RAPID1, ACR20 response rates at week 24 for the CZP 200 mg ($n = 393$) (the dose used in clinical practice) and 400 mg ($n = 390$) groups were 58.8% and 60.8%, respectively, compared with 13.6% for the PBO ($n = 199$) group (Table 5) [7]. Differences were significant from week 1 and sustained to week 52 ($p < 0.001$). At week 52, mean radiographic progression from baseline was reduced in patients treated with both doses of CZP compared to PBO. In the CZP 200 mg + MTX group, 69% of patients had no radiographic progression compared to 52% of patients who received PBO [7]. Overall rates of AEs were 125.9 per 100 patient-years in the PBO group and 96.6 per 100 patient-years and 94.6 per 100 patient-years in the CZP 200 mg and 400 mg groups, respectively. Most of these were of only mild or moderate severity. In particular, the frequency of infections was similar between all three groups. No significant differences were observed between the 200 mg and 400 mg maintenance doses of CZP – hence the choice of the 200 mg fortnightly maintenance dose as the one to be used in clinical practice [7].

The RAPID2 trial showed similar results to RAPID1 at week 24 (Table 5). Serious infections, including five cases of tuberculosis, occurred more frequently with CZP than PBO [38].

The FAST4WARD study evaluated 220 RA patients who had failed at least one csDMARD prior to receiving CZP [39]. Patients were treated with CZP 400 mg ($n = 111$) or PBO ($n = 109$) every four weeks for 24 weeks. At week 24, ACR20 response rates were 45.5% for CZP versus

9.3% for PBO ($p < 0.001$) (Table 5). Again, differences occurred as early as week 1. Most AEs were mild or moderate and no deaths or cases of TB were observed [39]. Injection site reactions occurred in 13.8% and 4.5% of CZP and PBO patients, respectively. Nine (8.1%) patients developed ADAb to CZP.

Another trial evaluated 247 patients who had active RA for at least six months despite MTX [40]. Patients received CZP 400 mg every four weeks for 24 weeks without a loading dose, in combination with MTX. The ACR20 response rates were 45.9% versus 22.9% for CZP + MTX (n = 126) and PBO + MTX (n = 121), respectively ($p < 0.001$) with improvement occurring from Week 1 in those who received CZP (Table 5) [40]. Infections occurred in 26.6% and 14.3% of patients in the CZP + MTX and PBO + MTX groups, respectively ($p = 0.026$). Of note, ADAb to CZP were reported in 5.0% of patients, which was lower than that reported in the FAST4WARD trial (8.1%) [39]. This may have been due to the protective effect of MTX co-administration.

***Certolizumab Pegol in csDMARD-Naïve Patients***

The efficacy and safety of CZP was assessed in csDMARD-naïve RA patients diagnosed within one year in a randomised, PBO-controlled, double-blind trial (C-EARLY) [10]. At baseline, 77.8% of subjects had radiographic erosions, indicating that most subjects already had radiographic progression even in "early" disease. Patients had a mean time since diagnosis at baseline of 2.9 months and were DMARD-naïve (including for MTX). Certolizumab pegol or PBO was administered SC in combination with MTX ($\geq$15 and $\leq$ 25 mg/week). Patients were treated with a loading dose of CZP 400 mg at week 0, 2 and 4 or PBO followed by 200 mg of CZP or PBO every two weeks for 52 weeks.

At week 52, more patients receiving CZP + MTX (n = 655) compared with PBO + MTX (n = 213) achieved sustained remission (DAS-28 erythrocyte sedimentation rate [DAS-28-ESR] < 2.6; 28.9% versus 15.0%, $p < 0.001$) and sustained LDA (43.8% versus 28.6%, $p < 0.001$) (Table 5)

[10]. Inhibition of radiographic progression and improvement in physical function were significantly greater for CZP + MTX versus PBO + MTX. Despite the relatively "aggressive" use of CZP in early RA, the incidence of AEs was similar in both groups [10].

### *Certolizumab Pegol versus Adalimumab*

The EXXELERATE trial was a 104-week randomised, single-blind (double blind until week 12 and investigator blind thereafter), head-to-head superiority study comparing CZP with ADL, both in combination with MTX [41]. Overall, 457 RA patients were randomised to CZP + MTX and 458 to ADL + MTX. No statistically significant difference was observed in ACR20 responses at week 12 (314/454, 69% patients and 324/454, 71% of patients; odds ratio [OR] 0·90 [95% CI 0·67–1·20]; p = 0·467) or DAS-28-ESR LDA at week 104 (161/454, 35% of patients and 152/454, 33% of patients; OR 1·09 [0·82–1·45]; p = 0·532) between CZP + MTX and ADL + MTX, respectively [41]. At week 12, 65 primary non-responders to CZP were switched to ADL and 57 primary non-responders to ADL were switched to CZP. Interestingly, despite both CZP and ADL being TNFi's, 33/57 (58%) of patients switching to CZP and 40/65 (62%) of patients switching to ADL responded 12 weeks later by achieving LDA or a DAS-28-ESR reduction ≥ 1·2 [41]. More studies are needed to determine why patients who fail one TNFi respond to another TNFi. There was a similar rate of infections in both groups.

### *Safety in Breastfeeding*

Reassuringly, the recent CRADLE study found no/minimal CZP transfer from plasma to breast milk occurred in 18 nursing mothers treated with CZP (either CZP 200 mg every 2 weeks or CZP 400 mg every 4 weeks) [42]. This suggests that continuation of CZP can occur during breast-feeding.

**Table 5. Key clinical trials involving certolizumab pegol**

| Study | Time of primary efficacy end-point | Responses | Proportion (%) of patients in each group for each response measure | | | | | |
|---|---|---|---|---|---|---|---|---|
| | | | PBO + MTX | PBO alone | CZP (200 mg q2w) + MTX | CZP (400 mg q2w) + MTX | CZP (400 mg q4w) | CZP (400 mg q4w) + MTX |
| RAPID 1 [7] | Week 24 | ACR20 | 13.6 | | 58.8 | 60.8 | | |
| | Week 24 | ACR50 | 8 | | 37 | 39.9 | | |
| RAPID 2 [38] | Week 24 | ACR20 | 8.7 | | 57.3 | 57.6 | | |
| | Week 24 | ACR50 | 3.1 | | 32.5 | 33.1 | | |
| FAST4WARD [39] | Week 24 | ACR20 | | 9.3 | | | 45.5 | |
| | Week 24 | ACR50 | | 3.7 | | | 22.7 | |
| Choy, 2012 [40] | Week 24 | ACR20 | 22.9 | | | | | 45.9 |
| | Week 24 | ACR50 | 5.9 | | | | | 18 |
| C-EARLY [10] | Week 52 | DAS-28 ESR < 2.6 | 15 | | 28.9 | | | |
| | Week 52 | ACR50 | 56.2 | | 61.8 | | | |

ACR20 = American College of Rheumatology criteria 20% improvement, ACR50 = American College of Rheumatology criteria 50% improvement, DAS-28 ESR = Disease activity score 28-joint count erythrocyte sedimentation rate, CZP = certolizumab pegol, PBO = placebo, MTX = methotrexate, q2w = every two weeks; q4w = every 4 weeks.

### Summary

Certolizumab pegol is an effective and well-tolerated TNFi in combination with MTX for the treatment of RA. The lack of an Fc component means it does not traverse the placenta. As it seems not to be excreted in breast milk [42], CZP appears to be the bDMARD of choice in the setting of pregnancy and breast-feeding. Although early use in csDMARD-naïve patients may be difficult under most national regulatory environments, such use in combination with MTX appears an effective and well-tolerated strategy to obtain sustained disease remission [41].

## GOLIMUMAB

### Mechanism of Action

Golimumab (GOL) is a human anti-TNF mAb that inhibits TNF activity by binding with high affinity and specificity to soluble and transmembrane TNF, thereby preventing ligand binding to its receptors [43].

### Clinical Trials

#### *Use in MTX Inadequate Responders (GO-FORWARD)*

Patients with active RA despite MTX were randomised to PBO + MTX (group 1, n = 133) and GOL administered SC every four weeks in the following groups: GOL 100 mg + PBO (group 2, n = 133), GOL 50 mg + MTX (group 3, n = 89), or GOL 100 mg + MTX (group 4, n = 89) [44]. Overall, ACR responses were consistently greater for GOL + MTX than MTX or GOL monotherapy at week 14 (time of primary end-point) and 24 with no difference in efficacy between the two GOL doses when used with MTX (Table 6). There was no significant difference in rate of

AEs, especially infections between groups. Interestingly, 92 patients (20.7%) had latent tuberculosis (TB) but study enrolment was allowed so long as treatment for this (usually isoniazid) was commenced. Reassuringly, none of these patients developed active TB despite immunosuppression. (However, this was in the context of close monitoring within a clinical trial). Five of 236 patients (2.1%) had ADAb at week 24 – all in the GOL monotherapy group [44].

Responses achieved at week 24 were sustained to week 52 [45]. However, those receiving GOL 100 mg + MTX (group 4) had an increased risk of serious AEs, especially serious infections (10 events per 100 patient-years, 95%CI 5-18) compared to those receiving MTX alone (2 events per 100 patient years, 95%CI 0 to 10) [45].

At week 252 (five years), 313 of the 444 patients (70.5%) randomised continued GOL with no new AE signals [46]. Overall, 429 GOL-treated patients had ≥ 1 blood sample taken. Of these patients, 32 (7.5%) tested positive for ADAbs to GOL and 25 of these (86.2%) were neutralising ADAbs [46]. However, this did not appear to impact the proportion of patients who discontinued GOL because of an AE or lack of efficacy.

### *Use in TNFi Failures (GO-AFTER)*

In this study, 461 patients with active RA despite a previous TNFi were randomised to receive SC injections of PBO (n = 155), GOL 50 mg (n = 153), or GOL 100 mg (n = 153) every four weeks [47]. Overall, 28 (18%) patients on PBO, 54 (35%) patients on GOL 50 mg (OR 2·5 [95%CI 1·5–4·2], p = 0·0006), and 58 (38%) patients on GOL 100 mg (2·8 [95%CI 1·6–4·7], p = 0·0001) achieved ACR20 responses at week 14. For weeks 1–16, serious AEs were recorded in 11 (7%) patients on PBO, 8 (5%) on GOL 50 mg and 4 (3%) on GOL 100 mg [47]. More patients in the two GOL groups achieved ACR20/50 responses than those receiving PBO (Table 6). There was no difference in efficacy between the two doses of GOL used. Forty-six percent of patients on PBO and 27% on GOL 50 mg received rescue therapy of an increased drug dose at week 16 while 2 (27%) of patients on GOL 100 mg met criteria for rescue therapy at week 16, but their GOL dose was not changed. Anti-drug antibodies to GOL were detected in only 8/264 (3%) patients who had blood samples taken at week 24. No new safety signals were detected at five years of follow-up while the cumulative incidence of ADAb at week 268 was low at 8.0% [48].

## Summary

Although it was the latest TNFi on the market, GOL's SC route of administration and dosing frequency of every four weeks is attractive. A recent report used data from the Canadian private and public drug databases of Ontario and Quebec and found the proportion of adherent (mean possession ratio ≥ 80%) patients in the GOL cohort (n = 595/683, 87%, $p < 0.0001$) was greater than in the groups receiving ADL (n = 1044/1400, 75%), ETN (n = 1285/1765, 73%) or CZP (132/187, 71%) [49]. This may have been due to the less frequent dosing schedule.

**Table 6. Key clinical trials involving golimumab**

| Study | Time of primary efficacy end-point | Responses | Proportion (%) of patients in each group for each response measure | | | | |
|---|---|---|---|---|---|---|---|
| | | | PBO + MTX | PBO alone | GOL alone | GOL + PBO | GOL + MTX |
| GO-FORWARD [44] | Week 14 | ACR20 | 33.1 | | | 44.4 | 55.6 |
| | Week 14 | ACR50 | 9.8 | | | 20.3 | 32 |
| GO-AFTER [47] | Week 14 | ACR20 | | 18 | 37 | | |
| | Week 14 | ACR50 | | 6 | 18 | | |

ACR20 = American College of Rheumatology criteria 20% improvement, ACR50 = American College of Rheumatology criteria 50% improvement, GOL = golimumab, PBO = placebo, MTX = methotrexate.

# TOCILIZUMAB

## Mechanism of Action

Tocilizumab (TCZ) is a humanised anti-IL-6R mAb that prevents IL-6 binding to both soluble and membrane-bound IL-6R. The importance of IL-6 blockade as a therapeutic strategy in the treatment of RA has long been recognised due to the widespread expression and pleiotropic nature of IL-6, which induces B- and T-lymphocyte proliferation and differentiation, and the differentiation of macrophages, osteoclasts, and megakaryocytes [50, 51].

## Clinical Trials

### *Use in Patients with an Inadequate Response to csDMARD or MTX*

#### The OPTION Trial (TCZ + MTX) [52]

In this double-blind, randomised, controlled trial, RA patients with an inadequate response to MTX were randomised to one of the following three groups: TCZ 8 mg/kg IV (n = 205), TCZ 4 mg/kg IV (n = 213), or PBO (n = 204) every four weeks for 24 weeks [52]. All three groups received MTX (10-25 mg weekly) throughout the study, while all other csDMARDS were discontinued at study entry. Approximately 55% and 66%% of patients received concomitant corticosteroids or NSAIDs, respectively.

The ACR20 responses were 59%, 48% and 26%, respectively ($p < 0.0001$ compared to PBO) while ACR50 responses were 44%, 31% and 11%, respectively ($p < 0.0001$ compared to PBO) (Table 7) [52]. Generally, TCZ 8 mg/kg provided a more frequent and stronger therapeutic effect than the 4 mg/kg dose.

There was no difference in serious AEs between groups, although a slightly higher risk of infection was noted in the two TCZ groups (21-31%) versus placebo (27%). Total cholesterol levels rose by 0.9 mmol/l, high-density lipoprotein cholesterol (HDL-C) levels rose by 0.1 mmol/l and low-density lipoprotein cholesterol (LDL-C) levels increased by 0.5-0.6 mmol/l in both TCZ groups with little change to these parameters in the PBO arm [52].

**The TOWARD Trial (TCZ + csDMARD) [5]**

In this double-blind, randomized controlled trial 1220 patients with an inadequate response to a csDMARD (MTX, HCQ, SSZ, LFN, AZA, or IM gold) remained on a stable dose of the csDMARD and received either TCZ 8 mg/kg IV (n = 805) or PBO (n = 415) every four weeks for 24 weeks [5]. The ACR20 responses at the primary end-point of week 24 were 60.8% and 24.5%, respectively with ACR50 responses of 37.6% and 9%, respectively (both $p < 0.0001$) (Table 7) [5].

The incidence of AEs was 72.8% in the TCZ + csDMARD group and 61.1% in the PBO + csDMARD group. Infection rates were 120.1 and 95.3 per 100 patient-years in the TCZ and PBO groups, respectively. The proportion of patients reporting serious AEs and serious infections in the TCZ versus PBO groups were 6.7% and 2.7% compared to 4.3% and 1.9%, respectively [5]. Neutropenia was noted more frequently in the TCZ group but there was no association between neutropenia and infection-related AEs. While the mechanism of neutropenia following TCZ administration remains unclear, TCZ does not appear to affect neutrophil apoptosis, phagocytosis or function [53]. None of the patients with grade 3 neutropenia (1,000–500 cells/mm$^3$) had to discontinue TCZ because of this. Tocilizumab was more commonly associated with elevation of alanine aminotransferase (ALT)/aspartate aminotransferase (AST) levels (< 3-fold the upper limit of normal) at some point during the study, but this was not associated with clinical features of hepatic dysfunction. Increases in mean fasting plasma lipid levels (within the normal range) were observed in the TCZ group only and were seen from week 6 onwards. Levels remained elevated throughout the study, with mean changes from baseline at week 24 as follows: total cholesterol + 0.8 mmol/L, HDL-C + 0.1 mmol/L and LDL-C + 0.5 mmol/L. The hyperlipidaemia responded to a statin in 16 patients who were commenced on this as per local guidelines [5].

**The LITHE Trial (TCZ + MTX, Radiographic and Functional Outcomes) [54]**

In this randomised, double-blind, PBO-controlled trial, patients with inadequate response to MTX (10-25 mg weekly) were randomised to one of three treatment arms: TCZ 8 mg/kg IV + MTX (n = 398), TCZ 4 mg/kg IV + MTX (n = 399), or PBO + MTX (n = 393) [54]. Unlike most of the other studies involving TCZ, primary end-points were not composite clinical measures but radiographic change from baseline as measured by the total Genant-modified Sharp Score (GmSS) and physical function as measured by area under the curve (AUC) of the Health Assessment Questionnaire Disability Index (HAQ-DI) at week 52. Changes in mean joint erosion, joint space narrowing and total GmSS showed significant differences from baseline in both TCZ + MTX groups compared to PBO + MTX, with greater protective benefit in the TCZ 8 mg/kg + MTX arm [54]. This is consistent with the known role of IL-6 in animal models of inflammatory arthritis as an important regulator of T-lymphocyte production of key osteoclastogenic cytokines and inflammation-induced bone marrow osteoclast differentiation [51]. An improvement in physical function as measured by the HAQ-DI was also noted [54].

The safety profile of TCZ was similar to that seen in other TCZ studies. Infections were the most common AE with a rate of 4.0, 3.7 and 2.3 per 100 patient-years for the TCZ 8 mg/kg IV + MTX, TCZ 4 mg/kg IV + MTX and PBO + MTX groups, respectively. As in the other studies, mean serum concentrations of total cholesterol, LDL-C, HDL-C, and triglycerides increased over time in those who received TCZ.

***Use in MTX-Naïve/MTX-Free Patients (AMBITION Trial [55])***

In this double-blind trial, patients with moderate-to-severe RA were randomised to receive TCZ 8 mg/kg IV monotherapy every 4 weeks or an escalating MTX dose of 7.5-20 mg weekly as monotherapy for 24 weeks [55]. All other csDMARDS were withdrawn prior to randomisation. The primary end-point of this study was to assess non-inferiority of TCZ compared to MTX for ACR20 response rates at week 24.

The ACR20 response rate for MTX (n = 284) was 52.5% versus 69.9% in the TCZ group (n = 286), while ACR50 responses were 33.5% versus 44.1% (p = 0.002), respectively (Table 7) [55]. Mean CRP levels normalised as early as week 2 following IV TCZ, and remained normal from week 12 to 24 in more than 90% of patients. Improvement in haemoglobin (Hb) levels was seen as early as week 2, with normalisation of mean Hb by week 6 in TCZ-treated patients. This was not seen with MTX.

The incidence of AEs for the TCZ group was 79.9% and 77.5% for MTX [55]. Adverse events which led to patient withdrawals were higher in the MTX group (5.3%) compared to TCZ (3.8%). Serious AEs (SAEs) and serious infections were higher in the TCZ group (SAEs 3.8%, infections 1.4%) compared to MTX (SAEs 2.8%, infections 0.7%) [55]. However, there was no association between the severity/frequency of infection and neutropenia in those who received TCZ.

### *Use in TNFi-Inadequate Responders*

#### The RADIATE Trial (TCZ + MTX) [56]

In this double-blind, randomised controlled trial, RA patients with an inadequate response to one or more TNFi's were randomised to one of the following three arms: TCZ 8 mg/kg IV + MTX (n = 175), TCZ 4 mg/kg IV + MTX, (n = 163) or PBO + MTX (n = 160), given every four weeks for 24 weeks [56]. The ACR20 responses were 50%, 30.4% and 10.1%, respectively, with ACR50 responses of 28.8%, 16.8% and 3.8%, respectively (Table 7) [56]. Similar results were observed regardless of the type or number of previously failed TNFi's.

Serious AEs were more common in the PBO + MTX group (11.3%) than the TCZ 8 mg/kg + MTX (6.3%) or TCZ 4 mg/kg + MTX (7.4%) groups. However, neutropenia and elevated HDL-C/LDL-C levels were commoner in those who received TCZ. In particular, 49 patients (28.0%), 33 patients (20.3%) and one patient (1.0%) in the 8 mg/kg, 4 mg/kg and PBO groups, respectively, had transient neutropenia at some time during the study. Although a higher proportion of patients experienced gastrointestinal (GI) AEs in the 8 mg/kg group, only two patients in each treatment group had serious GI AEs [56]. One patient in the 8 mg/kg group with a past history of diverticulosis suffered an acute diverticular perforation five days following the second infusion, but recovered fully. The authors concluded that as TCZ may suppress inflammatory symptoms and ESR/CRP and delay detection of diverticulitis, patients with a history of diverticulitis should be carefully observed during treatment with TCZ [56].

### *Tocilizumab versus Adalimumab Monotherapy*

#### The ADACTA Study [57]

This randomised, double-blind study compared TCZ monotherapy with ADL monotherapy in patients with RA and was the first study comparing two anti-cytokine agents as monotherapy [57]. Patients were randomised to receive TCZ 8 mg/kg IV (n = 162) every four weeks + PBO SC every two weeks or ADL 40 mg SC (n = 163) every two weeks + PBO IV every four weeks for 24 weeks. The mean change from baseline in DAS28 at week 24 was greater in the TCZ group (–3·3) than in the ADL group (–1·8) (difference –1·5, 95% CI –1·8 to –1·1; $p < 0{\cdot}0001$) [57]. More patients who received TCZ than ADL achieved Simplified Disease Activity Index (SDAI) remission at week 24 (30/163, 18·4% versus 13/162, 8·0%; $p < 0{\cdot}0067$). The TCZ group also had superior ACR responses (Table 7).

Serious AEs were similar between the two groups, although as seen in previous TCZ studies, more patients who received TCZ had higher serum LDL-C levels, increased ALT results, and lower platelet and neutrophil counts in the peripheral blood [57].

## Subcutaneous TCZ

Until recently, a limitation of TCZ was the inconvenience and cost of an IV infusion every four weeks. However, recent availability of a SC formulation has addressed this.

The SUMMACTA study enrolled 1262 patients with moderate-to-severe RA with an inadequate response to csDMARDS and demonstrated comparable efficacy (non-inferiority) of the SC formulation of TCZ 162 mg weekly compared to IV TCZ 8 mg/kg every four weeks [14]. As seen in previous TCZ studies, CRP fell in both groups immediately after the first dose of TCZ. A similar incidence of AEs was noted between the groups; except for injection site reactions, which were more common in the SC (10.1%) compared to the IV (2.4%) group [14]. Five patients in each group (0.8%) were positive for neutralising ADAb assays. This is important as a postulated explanation for the lower level of ADAb observed with IV TCZ was the lack of drug exposure to dendritic cells (specialist antigen presenting cells) present in subcutaneous tissue.

## Summary

Tocilizumab is a very effective bDMARD for the treatment of RA in combination with csDMARDS including MTX [5, 52] or as monotherapy [55]. It has a rapid onset of action within 2-4 weeks and appears superior to ADL as monotherapy [57]. The low level of ADAb with TCZ may at least partially explain its greater efficacy compared to ADL [14, 58]. Availability of a SC formulation provides a more convenient and less costly mode of administration compared to IV, although the need for a weekly (usually self-administered) SC dose may discourage some patients. Although longer-term studies are required, there is no evidence the observed hyperlipidaemia results in increased cardiovascular events [59]. A retrospective post-hoc analyses which pooled data from 3986 RA patients who received $>$ 1 dose of TCZ found an association between baseline total cholesterol: HDL-C ratio and an increased risk of cardiovascular events (acute myocardial infarction, stroke and cardiovascular death). However, the risk of cardiovascular events did not correlate with lipid profile changes while on TCZ treatment [60].

**Table 7. Key clinical trials involving tocilizumab**

| Study | Time of primary efficacy end-point | Responses | Proportion (%) of patients in each group for each response measure | | | | | | | | |
|---|---|---|---|---|---|---|---|---|---|---|---|
| | | | PBO + MTX | PBO alone | PBO + csDMARDS | MTX alone | ADL (40 mg) | TCZ (8 mg/kg) | TCZ (4 mg/kg) + MTX | TCZ (8 mg/kg) + MTX | TCZ (8 mg/kg) + cs DMARDS |
| OPTION [52] | Week 24 | ACR20 | 26 | | | | | | 48 | 59 | |
| | Week 24 | ACR50 | 11 | | | | | | 31 | 44 | |
| TOWARD [5] | Week 24 | ACR20 | | | 24.5 | | | | | | 60.8 |
| | Week 24 | ACR50 | | | 9 | | | | | | 37.6 |
| AMBITION [55] | Week 24 | ACR20 | | | | 52.5 | | 69.9 | | | |
| | Week 24 | ACR50 | | | | 33.5 | | 44.1 | | | |
| RADIATE [56] | Week 24 | ACR20 | 10.1 | | | | | | 30.4 | 50 | |
| | Week 24 | ACR50 | 3.8 | | | | | | 16.8 | 28.8 | |
| ADACTA [57] | Week 24 | ACR20 | | | | | 49.4 | 65 | | | |
| | Week 24 | ACR50 | | | | | 27.8 | 47.2 | | | |
| | Week 24 | Change in DAS28 | | | | | -1.8 | -3.3 | | | |

ACR20 = American College of Rheumatology criteria 20% improvement, ACR50 = American College of Rheumatology criteria 50% improvement, DAS28 = Disease activity score 28-joint count, ADL = adalimumab, TCZ = tocilizumab, csDMARDS = conventional synthetic disease modifying anti-rheumatic drugs, PBO = placebo, MTX = methotrexate.

The neutropenia seen during IL-6 blockade does not appear to correlate with an increased risk of infection. Dose reduction to 4 mg/kg (or even 6 mg/kg) may reduce the risk of AEs, e.g., abnormal liver function tests or neutropenia if concerned. However, this reduces efficacy (Table 7). Caution needs to be particularly exercised in those with a history of diverticular disease [56].

As IL-6 is a major driver of the acute phase response [50], the observed rapid lowering of acute phase reactants following TCZ administration is expected. However, as CRP is part of the acute phase response, CRP and perhaps ESR may be less reliable biomarkers of inflammation in a patient receiving TCZ. A corollary of this is that in the setting of IL-6 blockade, use of the SDAI rather than the DAS28 may be more appropriate, as there is a higher weighting of ESR/CRP with the latter outcome measure.

Interleukin-6 stimulates hepatic production of hepcidin, a protein which is part of the acute phase response and modulates Hb production by restricting iron availability [61]. Blockade of IL-6 has a marked inhibitory effect on hepatic hepcidin production, which leads to release of sequestered iron from macrophages and a rapid rise in haemoglobin. Tocilizumab is thus a very effective treatment for the anaemia of chronic disease seen in RA.

Other IL-6 blockading agents will soon be available. Sarilumab, a human IL-6R inhibitor, has completed phase 3 clinical trials [62] and appeared superior to ADL monotherapy [63]. Sirukumab, a monoclonal antibody that, unlike TCZ, inhibits the cytokine itself, is also in clinical trial [64]. The exact place of these newer agents in the treatment of RA and their advantages/disadvantages compared to TCZ remain unclear.

# ABATACEPT

## Mechanism of Action

Abatacept (ABA is a fusion protein of cytotoxic T lymphocyte-associated antigen-4 and immunoglobulin G1 that selectively modulates the CD80/CD86–CD28 co-stimulatory signal required for full T-lymphocyte activation [65].

## Clinical Trials

### *Use in MTX Inadequate Responders (AIM)*

The AIM study was a one-year multicentre trial in which patients with active RA despite MTX were randomised to ABA (10 mg/kg IV every four weeks, n = 433 patients) or PBO (n = 219 patients) [66]. At month 6, ACR20 and ACR50 responses were 67.9% for ABA versus 39.7% for PBO, and 39.9% for ABA versus 16.8% for PBO, respectively (Table 8). At month 12, the ACR20 and ACR50 responses increased to 73.1% for ABA versus 39.7% for PBO, and 48.3% for ABA versus 18.2% for PBO, respectively ($p < 0.001$ for all). At month 12, ABA-treated patients had approximately 50% reduction in change from baseline in GmSS compared with PBO [66].

There was a higher incidence of serious infections (2.5% vs. 0.9%) and infusion reactions (8.8% versus 4.1%) in the ABA-treated group compared to the PBO arm [66]. Six patients (1.4%) had ADAbs to ABA but this did not appear to affect efficacy.

### *Use in TNFi Inadequate Responders (ATTAIN and ARRIVE)*

The ATTAIN study randomised patients with active RA and an inadequate response to a TNFi to either ABA or PBO given on days 1, 15, and 29 and every 28 days thereafter for six months, in addition to at least one csDMARD [67]. At month 6, ACR20 responses were 50.4% in the ABA group and 19.5% in the PBO group ($p < 0.001$) while the rate of ACR50 responses was higher in those receiving ABA compared to PBO (20.3% versus 3.8%, $p < 0.001$) (Table 8) [67]. There was no difference in occurrence of serious infections between groups (2.3%) [67]. Anti-drug antibodies against ABA occurred in 3 of 234 (1.3%) patients.

The safety and efficacy of ABA was examined in a six-month open-label trial of 1046 RA patients who had failed a TNFi for three months or longer (ARRIVE) [8]. Patients were either switched to ABA directly (10 mg/kg IV on days 1, 15 and 29, and every 4 weeks thereafter) or after completing washout (discontinuation of TNFi for two months or longer). At six months, similar improvements were seen in disease activity as measured by DAS28–CRP, LDA, DAS28-defined remission, physical function and health-related quality of life in both groups of patients [8]. This suggested that direct switching from a TNFi to ABA was safe and effective.

### *Use in Early RA (AGREE)*

In this double-blind study, patients with RA for two years or less (mean of 6.5 months) were randomised to ABA 10 mg/kg IV (days 1, 15 and 29 and every 4 weeks thereafter) + MTX ($n = 256$) or PBO + MTX ($n = 253$) [68]. At month 12, a greater proportion of ABA + MTX-treated patients achieved DAS28-CRP defined remission (41.4% versus 23.3%; $p < 0.001$) (Table 8). Less radiographic progression was present in the ABA + MTX compared to the PBO + MTX groups (mean change in GmSS total score, 0.63 versus 1.06; $p = 0.040$). There was no difference in frequency of AEs between the two groups [68].

### *Use in Undifferentiated Inflammatory Arthritis or Very Early RA*

The effect of ABA on undifferentiated inflammatory arthritis (UA) or very early RA was investigated in ADJUST, a small double-blind PBO-controlled two-year study [69]. Patients who were anti-cyclic citrullinated peptide (CCP)2-positive with UA (clinical synovitis of two or more joints) but not fulfilling ACR criteria for RA were randomised to ABA (10 mg/kg, days 1, 15, 29, 57, 85, 113, 141 and 169) or PBO for six months. At month 12 (26 weeks following cessation of ABA), 12/26 (46%) of ABA-treated versus 16/24 (67%) of PBO-treated patients developed RA [69]. This suggested that ABA slowed progression of UA/very early RA in those at high risk of developing RA. A beneficial effect on radiographic and MRI progressive was also seen, which was maintained for six months following cessation of ABA [69]. This novel study suggested early T-lymphocyte modulation might have a beneficial effect on progression to RA.

***Ability to Sustain Remission Following Cessation (AVERT)***

In the AVERT study, patients with early active RA (mean duration of disease 6.7 months) were randomised to double-blind ABA 125 mg SC weekly + MTX, ABA 125 mg SC weekly monotherapy, or MTX for 12 months [15]. Patients with LDA (DAS28-CRP $< 3.2$) at month 12 entered a 12-month period of withdrawal of all RA therapy. For ABA + MTX versus MTX, DAS28-CRP $< 2.6$ (DAS remission) was achieved in 60.9% versus 45.2% ($p = 0.01$) of patients at 12 months. Combination ABA + MTX achieved higher rates of DAS remission compared to MTX alone following treatment withdrawal, in 14.8% versus 7.8% ($p = 0.045$), respectively at both month 12 and 18. In comparison, 12.4% of patients who received ABA monotherapy achieved DAS remission at both month 12 and 18. Both ABA groups had a similar safety profile to MTX alone [15].

The achievement of sustained drug-free remission following withdrawal of all RA therapy in a small number of patients suggested that early use of ABA might "re-set" the autoimmune process. This study also demonstrated the safety and effectiveness of the ABA SC formulation.

***Immunogenicity (ALLOW)***

In the ALLOW trial, following a 12-week open-label "run –in" phase (Period I: IV ABA loading dose 10 mg/kg and weekly SC ABA 125 mg), patients were randomised to double-blind SC PBO or SC ABA for 12 weeks (Period II). At the end of Period II, patients receiving SC ABA continued treatment and patients on PBO were re-introduced to SC ABA (12-week open-label period III) [16]. Immunogenicity to SC ABA was low, similar to that seen with IV ABA and unaffected by a three-month interruption and re-introduction of ABA [16].

### *Comparison with IFX (ATTEST)*

Patients with RA and an inadequate response to MTX were randomised to ABA (IV 10 mg/kg on days 1, 15 and 29, and every 28 days thereafter, n = 156), IFX (3 mg/kg IV on days 1, 15, 43 and 85, and every 56 days thereafter, n = 165), or PBO (every four weeks, n = 110) and background MTX [70].

At day 197, there was a greater fall in DAS28-ESR with ABA than PBO (-2.53 versus -1.48, $p < 0.001$). More patients entered DAS remission with ABA compared to PBO (11.3% versus 2.9%). Comparable efficacy was seen with IFX at this time-point. Similar differences between ABA and PBO were seen in ACR responses (Table 8).

At Day 365, for ABA versus IFX, reductions in the DAS28-ESR were –2.88 versus –2.25 with ACR20 response rates of 72.4% and 55.8% (estimate of difference 95% CI = 5.5, 27.8) and ACR50 response rates of 45.5 and 36.4% (estimate of difference 95% CI = –2.2, 20.5), respectively [70]. Disease Activity Score-28-defined remission occurred in 18.7 and 12.2%, respectively, of those receiving ABA and IFX [70].

Over 52 weeks, serious AEs occurred in 9.6 versus 18.2%, of those receiving ABA compared to IFX, with serious infections occurring in 1.9 versus 8.5% of those receiving ABA or IFX, respectively [70].

While one might consider the use of IFX 3 mg/kg every eight weeks as a relatively low dose, ABA was at least as effective as this dose and had better tolerability and safety than even this low dose of IFX.

### *Comparison with ADL (AMPLE)*

Patients with active RA and an inadequate response to MTX were randomised to ABA 125 mg SC weekly + MTX or ADL 40 mg SC fortnightly + MTX [13]. At month 12, there was a similar ACR20 response rate between the groups (64.8% of patients in the ABA group and 63.4% in the ADL group) with a similar rate of radiographic non-progression between groups (Table 8). Injection site reactions occurred in 3.8% of those taking ABA compared to 9.1% of those receiving ADL ($p = 0.006$) but there was no difference in infection rates [13].

Fewer patients receiving ABA developed a positive ANA (5.2%) compared to 13.3% of those taking ADL. Fewer patients on ABA (0.3%) developed a positive dsDNA titre compared to 9.9% of those receiving ADL [13].

The two-year data from AMPLE demonstrated sustained and comparable therapeutic efficacy for ABA and ADL [13]. However, there were fewer SAEs and fewer discontinuations due to AEs or SAEs in the ABA group. In particular, serious infections occurred in 3.8% (n = 12 patients) of ABA patients versus 5.8% (n = 19 patients) of those receiving ADL. None of the serious infections in the ABA group led to treatment discontinuation, nine of the 19 serious infections led to discontinuation of ADL.

## Abatacept and Malignancy

Interestingly, while ABA down-regulates T-lymphocyte co-stimulation, the opposite strategy of up-regulating T-lymphocyte co-stimulation with novel agents such as ipilimumab has revolutionized the treatment of melanoma and other solid organ malignancies [71].

While this raises theoretical concern ABA might be oncogenic, a recently published systematic review and meta-analysis showed no increased risk of malignancy with ABA compared to csDMARDS or PBO [72]. Comparison of 4134 RA patients treated with ABA in seven clinical trials and 41 529 csDMARD-treated RA patients from five observational cohorts also found no increased risk of malignancy or lymphoma with ABA [73]. A retrospective study of 9460 patients with RA or inflammatory bowel disease who commenced MTX or bDMARDS after a non-melanomatous skin cancer (NMSC) showed that ABA (hazard ratio 1.40, 95% CI 0.48-4.03) was not associated with an increased risk of another NMSC [74].

**Table 8. Key clinical trials involving abatacept**

| Study | Time of primary efficacy end-point | Responses | Proportion (%) of patients in each group for each response measure | | | | | |
|---|---|---|---|---|---|---|---|---|
| | | | PBO + MTX | PBO + csDMARDS | ADL + MTX | ABA + MTX | ABA + csDMARDS | IFX + MTX |
| AIM [66] | Month 6<br>Month 6 | ACR20<br>ACR50 | 39.7<br>16.8 | | | 67.9<br>39.9 | | |
| ATTAIN [67] | Month 6<br>Month 6 | ACR20<br>ACR50 | | 19.5<br>3.8 | | | 50.4<br>20.3 | |
| AGREE [68] | Month 12<br>Month 12 | DAS28-CRP remission<br>ACR50 | 23.3<br>42.3 | | | 41.4<br>57.4 | | |
| ATTEST [70] | Day 197<br>Day 197 | ACR20<br>ACR50 | 41.8<br>20 | | | 66.7<br>40.4 | | 59.4<br>37 |
| AMPLE [13] | Month 12<br>Month 12 | ACR20<br>ACR50 | | | 63.4<br>46 | 64.8<br>46.2 | | |

ACR20 = American College of Rheumatology criteria 20% improvement, ACR50 = American College of Rheumatology criteria 50% improvement, DAS28-CRP = Disease activity score 28-joint count C-reactive protein, ABA = abatacept, ADL = adalimumab, csDMARDS = conventional synthetic disease modifying anti-rheumatic drugs, IFX = infliximab, PBO = placebo, MTX = methotrexate.

## Summary

Abatacept is an effective treatment for RA in combination with MTX. It appears at least as effective as either IFX (3 mg/kg every eight weeks) [70] or ADL [13] and is better tolerated with a lower risk of serious infection than either of these TNFi's. There is intriguing data suggesting it may have a role in preventing evolution of early UA into RA [15, 69]. It appears less likely to induce ANA or dsDNA than a TNFi [13].

# RITUXIMAB

## Mechanism of Action

Rituximab (RTX) is a chimeric mouse-human mAb against CD20 that selectively depletes B-lymphocytes by several mechanisms including antibody-dependent cell-mediated cytotoxicity, complement-dependent cytotoxicity, and promotion of CD20 B-cell apoptosis [75-77]. The CD20 surface marker is expressed on B-cells but not stem cells or plasma cells.

## Clinical Trials

### *Use in Early RA (IMAGE)*

The IMAGE trial was a randomised, double-blind, PBO-controlled, multi-center study that randomised 755 MTX-naïve patients with early active RA to RTX (500 mg or 1000 mg given on days 1 and 15) + MTX (initiated at 7.5 mg/week and increased to 20 mg/week by week 8) compared to MTX alone [78]. At week 52, only patients in the RTX 1000 mg (n = 251) and not the RTX 500 mg (n = 252) group met the primary end-point of reduction in radiographic damage using the GmSS compared to patients who received MTX alone. The ACR responses are shown in Table 9. Frequency of AEs was similar between treatment groups [78].

***Use in MTX-Inadequate Responders (SERENE and DANCER)***

The SERENE trial randomised 509 bDMARD-naïve RA patients with active RA despite MTX to RTX 500 mg (two infusions, n = 168) + MTX or 1000 mg (two infusions, n = 172) + MTX or PBO (n = 172) + MTX [79]. During weeks 16 to 23, patients were allowed "rescue" therapy of one additional csDMARD. This was given to 9.3% of the PBO group, 3.6% of the RTX 500 mg group, and 2.3% of the RTX 1000 mg group. From week 24, those patients not in DAS remission (DAS28 < 2.6) received a second course of RTX while those who initially received PBO were switched to RTX 500 mg (two infusions). At week 24, both RTX groups had better responses compared to PBO ($p < 0.0001$) with ACR20 responses of 54%, 51% and 23% for RTX 500 mg + MTX, RTX 1000 mg + MTX and PBO + MTX, respectively (Table 9) [79]. Further improvements were seen in both RTX arms from week 24 to week 48. The incidence of AEs was comparable between all three groups. The most common AEs were infusion-related reactions, RA flares, nasopharyngitis, and upper respiratory tract infections. At week 24, positive human anti-chimeric antibodies (HACAs) were observed in 7.9%, 5.4% and 3.6% of those who received RTX 2×500 mg + MTX, RTX 2×1000 mg + MTX and PBO + MTX, respectively. No association was noted between the presence of HACAs and infusion-related reactions or secondary failure to RTX. Infusion-related reactions were more common in those receiving a first RTX infusion of 1000 mg (25%) compared with a first infusion of RTX 500 mg or PBO (19% and 14%, respectively) but were less common with subsequent infusions. Patients who were seropositive had better responses to RTX over time, especially at week 48, compared to those who were seronegative. No association was seen between low serum Ig levels and infections [79].

The DANCER trial was a randomised, double-blind, PBO-controlled, dose-ranging study in which 465 patients with moderate-to-severe RA and prior csDMARDS or bDMARDS other than MTX were treated with RTX 500 mg or 1000 mg, corticosteroids and ongoing MTX (10-25 mg/week) [80]. At week 24, more patients receiving RTX 500 mg or 1000 mg had ACR20 ($p \leq 0.001$), ACR50 ($p \leq 0.001$), and ACR70 ($p < 0.05$) responses compared to PBO (Table 9). There was no significant difference in the likelihood of an ACR20 response between the RTX 1000 mg and 500 mg dose [80]. Nearly complete depletion of peripheral blood B-cells occurred with RTX and persisted throughout the 24-week study period. Recovery of peripheral blood B-cells began after week 16. Overall, HACAs were detected in 0.7%, 4.2%, and 2.7% of the PBO, RTX 2 x 500 mg and RTX 2 x 1000 mg groups, respectively.

Adverse events were reported in 70%, 81%, and 85% of patients in the PBO, RTX 500 mg and RTX 1000 mg groups, respectively [80]. Most of these were mild-to-moderate. The commonest AEs were headache, nausea, and upper respiratory tract infections (URTIs). Infections (mainly URTIs) occurred in 28% of those who received PBO compared to 35% of RTX-treated patients. Premedication with IV methylprednisolone reduced the incidence and severity of infusion-related reactions.

***Use in TNFi-Inadequate Responders (REFLEX)***

The REFLEX trial was a 2-year, multicentre, randomised, double-blind, PBO-controlled study in which patients with active RA and an inadequate response to ≥ 1 TNFi were randomised to IV RTX (2 infusions of 1000 mg each, n = 311 patients) or PBO (n = 209), both with background MTX [81]. At week 24, more ($p < 0.0001$) RTX-treated patients had ACR20 (51% versus 18%) and ACR50 (27% versus 5%) responses compared to those receiving PBO (Table 9) [81]. Over 90% of patients had received ≤ 2 TNFi, with 9% having had three TNFi's. Thirteen patients (4.3%) had positive HACAs but there was no association between these and AEs or ACR responses. Although almost complete depletion of peripheral blood CD20+ B-lymphocytes occurred, mean Ig levels remained normal. Most AEs occurred with the first RTX infusion and were of mild-to-moderate severity. The rate of serious infections was 5.2 per 100 patient-years in the RTX group compared to 3.7 per 100 patient-years in those receiving PBO [81].

**Table 9. Key clinical trials involving rituximab**

| Study | Time of primary efficacy end-point | Responses | Proportion (%) of patients in each group for each response measure | | | | | |
|---|---|---|---|---|---|---|---|---|
| | | | MTX alone | PBO alone | MTX + RTX (500 mg) | RTX (500 mg) | MTX + RTX (1000 mg) | RTX (1000 mg) |
| IMAGE [78] | Week 52 | ACR20 | 64.3 | | 76.7 | | 80 | |
| | Week 52 | ACR50 | 41.8 | | 59.4 | | 64.8 | |
| SERENE [79] | Week 24 | ACR20 | 23.3 | | 54.5 | | 50.6 | |
| | Week 24 | ACR50 | 9.3 | | 26.3 | | 25.9 | |
| DANCER [80] | Week 24 | ACR20 | | 28 | | 55 | | 54 |
| | Week 24 | ACR50 | | 13 | | 33 | | 34 |
| REFLEX [81] | Week 24 | ACR20 | | 18 | | | | 51 |
| | Week 24 | ACR50 | | 5 | | | | 27 |

ACR20 = American College of Rheumatology criteria 20% improvement, ACR50 = American College of Rheumatology criteria 50% improvement, PBO = placebo, MTX = methotrexate, RTX = rituximab.

## Summary

Rituximab is an effective and well-tolerated treatment for RA – even in those who have failed ≥ 1 TNFi. Seropositive patients appeared to have better responses to RTX [79]. Although similar clinical responses occur for both RTX doses, only the 2×1000 mg dose significantly slowed progression of joint damage [78]. While persistent B-lymphocyte depletion occurs following RTX, this did not appear to significantly increase the risk of infection. As RTX has been used for many years in the treatment of lymphoma, many rheumatologists are comfortable using it in the setting of previous malignancy.

# TOFACITINIB

## Mechanism of ACTION

Tofacitinib (TFN) is a selective oral inhibitor of the Janus kinase (JAK) family of kinases which particularly inhibits JAK3 and/or JAK1 [82]. This blocks signalling through the common gamma chain which contains receptors for several cytokines, including IL-2, -4, -7, -9, -15, and -21, which are important in lymphocyte activation, proliferation and function [83]. Inhibition of JAK1 also modulates signalling by pro-inflammatory cytokines, such as IL-6 and the interferons [84].

## Clinical Trials

### *Use as Monotherapy (ORAL SOLO)*

In this double-blind, PBO-controlled study, 611 patients with active RA were randomised to oral TFN 5 mg twice daily (bd), TFN 10 mg bd or PBO for three months followed by TFN 5 mg bd or PBO for three months followed by TFN 10 mg bd [9]. At month 3, more patients receiving TFN achieved ACR20 responses (59.8% in the TFN 5 mg bd and 65.7% in the

TFN 10 mg bd groups, compared to 26.7% in the PBO group, $p < 0.001$ for both comparisons) (Table 10) [9]. Serious infections developed in six patients who received TFN. Common AEs were headache and URTI. Mean LDL-C levels increased by 3.5% with PBO, 13.6% with TFN 5 mg BD and 19.1% with TFN 10 mg BD. Neutropenia occurred more frequently among those receiving TFN, but no serious infections were noted in those with moderate-to-severe neutropenia [9]. (Interestingly, raised LDL-C and neutropenia have also been noted in the TCZ clinical trials – see above).

***Compared to MTX (ORAL START)***

In this trial, MTX-naive RA patients ($n = 958$) were randomised to TFN 5 mg bd or TFN 10 mg bd or MTX $\leq$ 20 mg/week as monotherapy [85]. Mean changes in mTSS from baseline to month 6 were less in those receiving TFN compared to MTX, but these changes were mild (0.2 points in the TFN 5 mg bd group and < 0.1 point in the TFN 10 mg bd group compared to 0.8 points in the MTX group, $p < 0.001$ for both comparisons. (The minimal clinically important difference in mTSS is 4.6 points [86]). Radiographic outcomes were similar between the two TFN groups even at 24 months. (Interestingly, the authors chose ACR70 rather than the more usual ACR20/50 as one of the primary end-points). Among those who received TFN, 25.5% in the 5 mg bd group and 37.7% in the TFN 10 mg bd group had ACR70 responses at month 6 compared to 12.0% of those who received MTX ($p < 0.001$ for both comparisons) (Table 10) [85]. Herpes zoster developed in 31/770 (4.0%) patients who received TFN compared to 2/186 (1.1%) who received MTX. Tofacitinib was associated with a mild increase in creatinine and LDL-C/HDL-C levels.

***Use in Combination with csDMARDS (ORAL-SYNC)***

This double-blind trial randomised 792 patients with active RA despite csDMARDS (mostly MTX) to TFN 5 mg bd or 10 mg bd, or PBO, which was then subsequently switched at month 3 to TFN 5 mg bd or TFN 10 mg bd [87]. At month 6, ACR20 response rates for the 5 mg bd and 10 mg bd TFN groups were 52.1% and 56.6%, respectively, compared to 30.8% in the PBO group (Table 10). Incidence rates of serious AEs for patients receiving TFN 5 mg bd, TFN 10 mg bd, or PBO were 6.9, 7.3, or 10.9 events per 100 patient-years of exposure, respectively [87]. During months 6-12, serious infections were only reported in the TFN 10 mg bd group. As seen in other SOLO trials, neutropenia and elevated LDL-C/HDL-C levels were noted in those receiving TFN.

### *Compared to Adalimumab (ORAL STANDARD and ORAL STRATEGY)*

In ORAL STANDARD, 717 patients with active RA despite MTX were randomised to TFN 5 mg bd, TFN 10 mg bd, ADL 40 mg every 2 weeks, or PBO [88]. At month 3, patients receiving PBO who did not have a 20% reduction from baseline in the number of swollen and tender joints were switched to either TFN 5 mg bd or 10 mg bd. At month 6, all patients still receiving PBO were switched to TFN. At month 6, ACR20 response rates were higher among those receiving TFN 5 mg bd or TFN 10 mg bd (51.5% and 52.6%, respectively) and those receiving ADL (47.2%) compared to those receiving PBO (28.3%) ($p < 0.001$ for all comparisons) (Table 10) [88]. Adverse events occurred more frequently with TFN than PBO, and pulmonary TB occurred in two patients receiving TFN 10 mg bd. Again, TFN was associated with an increase in LDL-C/HDL-C and neutropenia.

In ORAL STRATEGY, a double-blind, head-to-head, non-inferiority, randomised controlled trial, 1146 patients with active RA despite MTX were randomised to receive TFN 5 mg bd monotherapy (n = 384), TFN 5 mg bd + MTX (n = 376), or ADL 40 mg sc every other week + MTX (n = 386) [89]. At month 6, ACR50 responses were observed in 147/384 (38%) of patients who took TFN monotherapy, 173/376 (46%) of those who received TFN + MTX, and 169/386 (44%) of patients who received ADL + MTX (Table 10). Overall, TFN + MTX was non-inferior to ADL + MTX [89]. A similar frequency of AEs in the different treatment arms was noted. In particular, herpes zoster occurred in 18 patients (2%) overall; 4/384 (1%) in the TFN monotherapy group, 8/376 (2%) in the TFN + MTX group, and 6/386 (2%) of those in the ADL + MTX group [89].

**Table 10. Key clinical trials involving tofacitinib**

| Study | Time of primary efficacy end-point | Responses | Proportion (%) of patients in each group for each response measure | | | | | | |
|---|---|---|---|---|---|---|---|---|---|
| | | | PBO alone | MTX alone | TFN (5 mg) | TFN (10 mg) | TFN (5 mg) + MTX | ADL | ADL + MTX |
| ORAL SOLO [9] | Month 3<br>Month 3 | ACR20<br>ACR50 | 26.7<br>12.5 | | 59.8<br>31.1 | 65.7<br>36.5 | | | |
| ORAL START [85] | Month 6 | ACR70 | | 12 | 25.5 | 37.7 | | | |
| ORAL SYNC [87] | Month 6<br>Month 6 | ACR20<br>ACR50 | 30.8<br>12.6 | | 52.1<br>33.3 | 56.6<br>35.5 | | | |
| ORAL STANDARD [88] | Month 6 | ACR20 | 28.3 | | 51.5 | 52.6 | | 47.2 | |
| ORAL STRATEGY [89] | Month 6 | ACR50 | | | 38 | | 46 | | 44 |
| ORAL STEP [90] | Month 3<br>Month 3 | ACR20<br>ACR50 | 24.4<br>8.4 | | 41.7<br>26.5 | 48.1<br>27.8 | | | |

ACR20 = American College of Rheumatology criteria 20% improvement, ACR50 = American College of Rheumatology criteria 50% improvement, ACR70 = American College of Rheumatology criteria 70% improvement, ADL = adalimumab, PBO = placebo, MTX = methotrexate, TFN = tofacitinib.

***Use in TNFi Failures (ORAL STEP)***

In this double-blind, parallel-group study, 399 patients with active RA and an inadequate response to a TNFi were randomised to receive TFN 5 mg bd (n = 133), TFN 10 mg bd (n = 134), or PBO (n = 132), all with MTX [90]. Overall, 257/399 patients (64%) had previously received one TNFi, 104 (26%) had received two, and 32 (8%) had received three or more. At month 3, patients given PBO were switched to either TFN 5 mg bd (n = 66) or TFN 10 mg bd (n = 66). At month 3, ACR20 response rates were 41·7% (n = 55/132; p = 0·0024) for TFN 5 mg bd and 48·1% (n = 64/133; p < 0·0001) for TFN 10 mg bd, compared to 24·4% (n = 32/131) for PBO (Table 10) [90]. Time to an ACR20 response was two weeks for patients receiving either dose of TFN.

The commonest AEs in the first three months of treatment with TFN were diarrhoea (n = 13/267; 4·9%), nasopharyngitis (n = 11/267; 4·1%), headache (n = 11/267; 4·1%), and urinary tract infection (n = 8/267; 3·0%) [90].

## Tofacitinib and Herpes Zoster

Overall, 636 cases of herpes zoster (HZ) were reported in 6192 RA patients treated with TFN (incidence rate: 4.0 HZ events per 100 patient-years, 95% CI 3.7–4.4) in two phase I, nine phase II, six phase III, and two long-term extension studies of TFN in RA patients (16 839 patient-years, median time to first herpes zoster event 1.6 years) [91].

Most (93%) of the cases were “non-serious” and involved only one dermatome (94%). However, as these patients were enrolled in a clinical trial, most (570, 89.6%) were promptly commenced on anti-viral treatment. The incidence rates of HZ (number of unique patients with events per 100 patient-years) varied across regions, from 2.4 (95% CI 2.0–2.9) in Eastern Europe to 8.0 (95% CI 6.6–9.6) in Japan and 8.4 (95% CI 6.4–10.9) in Korea. The incidence rates were lowest for TFN 5 mg bd monotherapy without glucocorticoids (incidence rate: 0.56 [95% CI 0.07–2.01]) and highest for TFN 10 mg bd with csDMARDS and glucocorticoids (incidence rate: 5.44 [95% CI 3.72–7.68]). Overall, older age, glucocorticoid use, higher TFN dose and Asian geographic location were independent risk factors for HZ. Although the mechanism by which TFN increases the risk of HZ is unclear, its inhibitory effect on IFN signaling may be implicated [91].

### Summary

Tofacitinib is the first oral small molecule inhibitor for the treatment of RA and appears as effective as a TNFi [88, 89] and more effective as monotherapy than MTX [85]. The smaller dose of TFN 5 mg bd appears to be associated with a lower risk of infection and AEs than the TFN 10 mg bd dose. The oral route of administration makes it an attractive therapeutic option for those who are intolerant of a parenteral route of administration. The increased risk of herpes zoster may be an issue although most of the cases in the clinical trials were not serious [91].

## Baricitinib

Baricitinib is an oral inhibitor of JAK1 and JAK2, which has recently completed Phase 3 clinical trials. Although not yet licensed for the treatment of RA, it was effective in those who failed to respond to a range of csDMARDS [92] and bDMARDS [93], and appeared superior to ADL monotherapy [94]. The once daily dosing is more convenient than the bd dosing of TFN. Infections were more common in those receiving baricitinib compared to PBO [94]. Its exact place in therapy remains to be determined.

## BIOSIMILARS

A biosimilar is a biologic product with similar (but not identical), physicochemical characteristics and biologic activity, comparable pharmacokinetics and pharmacodynamics and similar safety, efficacy and clinical immunogenicity to the originator/reference/innovator molecule [95]. Expiry of patents protecting several originator molecules, which have resulted in large profits for their manufacturers, has led to the development of biosimilar drugs by competitors. This has been of great interest to governments and other funding bodies due to the cost of current bDMARDS.

While some have been reassuring about the use of biosimilars [96, 97], others have expressed caution that switching between a bDMARD and a biosimilar may increase immunogenicity (see later section on ADAb) – potentially compromising patient safety and drug efficacy [98-100].

The recently published Norwegian government-funded multicentre randomised, non-inferiority (pre-specified margin of 15%), double-blind trial (NOR-SWITCH) has been a helpful addition to the available evidence base [101]. Adult patients on stable treatment for inflammatory bowel disease, inflammatory arthritis or psoriasis with IFX originator for at least six months were randomised to either continue the IFX originator or switch to CT-P13 treatment (IFX biosimilar). Four hundred and eighty two patients were randomised (241 to IFX originator, 241 to CT-P13), while one patient was excluded from the full analysis and safety set for CT-P13 and 408 were included in the per-protocol analysis (202 in the IFX originator group and 206 in the CT-P13 group). One hundred and fifty five patients (32%) in the full analysis dataset had Crohn's disease, 93 (19%) had ulcerative colitis, 91 (19%) had spondyloarthritis, 77 (16%) had RA, 30 (6%) had psoriatic arthritis, and 35 (7%) had chronic plaque psoriasis. Disease worsening occurred in 26% (53/241) of patients in the IFX originator group and 30% (61/241) of those in the CT-P13 group (treatment difference 95% CI –12·7 to 3·9) [101]. There was a similar AE frequency between the groups [101]. No immunogenicity concerns were observed with similar serum drug concentrations and occurrence of ADAb between the two groups [101].

Another recent publication described a nationwide non-medical switch from originator IFX to CT-P13 in 802 Danish patients with RA, psoriatic arthritis and axial spondyloarthritis [102]. Disease activities were similar three months before and after the switch.

The PLANETRA study was a randomised, double-blind, multicentre, international study in which patients with active RA despite MTX were randomised to CT-P13 at a dose of 3 mg/kg (n = 302) or IFX originator (n = 304), both with MTX [6]. Therapeutic clinical equivalence was concluded if the 95% CI for the treatment difference in ACR20 responses was within 15% of each other. At week 30, ACR20 responses were 60.9% for CT-P13 and 58.6% for IFX (treatment difference 95% CI −6% to 10%) [6]. The incidence of drug-related AEs and presence of ADAb (48.4% for CT-P13 and 48.2% for IFX) were similar [6]. Overall, the IFX biosimilar CT-P13 appeared well-tolerated and effective compared to IFX originator. No additional safety signals were seen in the two-year extension study [6].

Another IFX biosimilar (SB2) has been studied [103]. Patients with moderate-to-severe RA despite MTX were randomised to either SB2 or IFX originator administered at weeks 0, 2 and 6 and every 8 weeks thereafter until week 46. At week 54, patients who previously received IFX originator were re-randomised to SB2 (IFX/SB2, n = 94 patients) or ongoing IFX originator (IFX/IFX, n = 101) until week 70. Those who previously received SB2 continued on SB2 (SB2/SB2, n = 201) until week 70. Efficacy, rates of infusion reaction and AEs were similar between treatment groups [103]. In particular, in those who were negative for ADAb up to week 54, newly developed ADAb occurred in 14.6%, 14.9% and 14.1% of the IFX/SB2, IFX/IFX and SB2/SB2 groups, respectively [103].

In a randomised, double-blind, multicentre study, patients with moderate-to-severe RA despite MTX were randomised to receive a weekly dose of SB4 50 mg sc (an ETN biosimilar) or ETN originator [104]. The ACR20 response rate at week 24 was 78.1% for SB4 and 80.3% for ETN (treatment difference 95% CI was −9.41 to 4.98%; within the pre-defined equivalence margin of −15% to 15%) [104]. This indicated therapeutic equivalence between SB4 and ETN. A similar rate of AEs was observed between the two groups and the incidence of ADAb up to week 24 was lower in SB4 compared with ETN (0.7% vs 13.1%, respectively) [104]. The 2-year extension study showed no loss of efficacy or increased immunogenicity when patients were switched from ETN to SB4 [105]. A recent study has also demonstrated equivalent efficacy between another ETN biosimilar (HD203) and ETN in RA [106].

### Summary

Despite initial concerns, ETN and IFX biosimilars had similar efficacy and tolerability to the originator molecule. However, no published study has examined the efficacy and safety of multiple switches between originator and biosimilar molecules or between two biosimilars in the treatment of inflammatory arthritis. As RA is a chronic disease, longer-term studies of biosimilars are required. Many uncertainties remain regarding the use and regulation of biosimilars. However, it is hoped the availability of biosimilars will lower the cost of treating patients and increase access to optimal bDMARD therapy for patients with inflammatory arthritis [107].

## Anti-Drug Antibodies (ADAb)

Although targeted blockade of TNF has been a major therapeutic advance in the treatment of inflammatory arthritis, a significant proportion of patients fail to respond to a TNFi (primary failure) or lose response over time (secondary failure). One possible mechanism for secondary failure is the development of neutralising ADAb. These have not been described with small molecule inhibitors such as TFN. Depending on the nature of the drug these may be HACA or human anti-human antibodies (HAHA) [108]. Binding of these antibodies to the TNFi or other bDMARD may result in immune complex formation, enhanced drug clearance and lower serum drug levels [109]. Alternatively, antibodies may neutralise the TNFi or other bDMARD by direct binding to the drug [110].

Free ADAbs in the serum are usually detected by either a classical sandwich ELISA or an antigen binding test where immunoglobulins from patient serum are aggregated on a protein (Sepharose) and ADAb is detected by a labelled therapeutic antibody [111]. The pH-shift anti-idiotype antigen-binding test (PIA) can be used to detect both bound and free ADAb, as lowering the pH will dissociate the ADAb-drug complex first before detection of the ADAb by an antigen binding test [112]. Assay variability, uncertainty regarding appropriate reference ranges for neutralising antibodies or serum drug levels, and variability in timing of blood sampling explains much of the variability in frequency of ADAb between different studies [108].

Despite being a fully humanised mAb, ADL often induces an immune response in patients [108]. A prospective cohort study of 272 RA patients found 76/272 (28%) developed ADL ADAb, mostly during the first 28 weeks of treatment. Those without ADAb had higher serum levels of ADL while those who developed ADAb were more likely to stop treatment due to treatment failure (HR 3.0, 95% CI 1.6-5.5; $p < 0.001$) [113]. More patients without ADAb had minimal disease activity compared to those with ADAb (n = 95/196, 48% versus n = 10/76, 13%) [113]. In other work, 407 TNFi-naïve RA patients were treated with ETN (n = 203) or ADL (n = 204). Fifty-four (26%) of the ADL-treated patients developed ADAb during treatment whereas ETN did not appear to generate ADAb [114]. While clinical response rates were similar for ETN and ADL, in the case of ADL this was strongly dependent on the presence or absence of ADL ADAb [114]. In that patient cohort, MTX appeared to reduce the development of ADL ADAb in a dose-dependent manner with MTX 22.5 mg/week being more effective than lower doses of MTX and MTX 10 mg/week being the lowest dose required to inhibit ADAb production [115].

Infliximab is a chimeric murine/human mAb and therefore potentially more immunogenic when infused into humans. Development of anti-IFX antibodies was associated with lower serum IFX trough levels, an increased risk of infusion reactions and treatment failure [116]. In 85 RA patients treated with IFX for a median of 4.4 (range 0.4-10.2) years, nine (10.5%); all of them with high levels of IFX ADAb, developed infusion-related reactions. These findings suggested the presence of ADAb was not only associated with poorer clinical response but also with infusion reactions. In the ATTRACT trial, HACA formation occurred in 53%, 21%, and 7% of those who received IFX at doses of 1, 3, and 10 mg/kg, respectively [117]. Concomitant administration of MTX with IFX at a dose of 7.5 mg/week reduced the development of HACA, with incidence rates of 15%, 7%, and 0% at IFX doses of 1, 3, and 10 mg/kg, respectively [117]. These data suggested immune tolerance to IFX occurred with higher IFX doses, especially in the presence of MTX [117]. Clinical response to both IFX and ADL was positively correlated with serum drug levels and inversely correlated with levels of ADAb against the corresponding TNFi [118].

A systematic review and meta-analysis of 17 clinical trials (one RCT and 16 observational studies) involving patients with inflammatory arthritis or inflammatory bowel disease concluded that clinical response was reduced by 68% (RR = 0.32, 95% CI = 0.22 to 0.48) in the presence of ADAb against IFX or ADL [119]. Interestingly, ADAb against ETN were not reported. Concomitant use of MTX or AZA/mercaptopurine appeared to reduce the likelihood of ADAb by 47% (RR = 0.53, 95% CI = 0.42 to 0.67) [119].

Unlike the above mAbs, CZP lacks an Fc region and therefore does not fix complement or cause antibody dependent cell mediated cytotoxicity *in vitro*. This may make it less immunogenic than a complete mAb and explain why ADAb to CZP were detected in only 6.4% of patients who received CZP + MTX in the RAPID1 trial [7] and 5.1% of patients who received CZP + MTX in the RAPID2 trial [38].

Etanercept is a fusion protein of two TNF receptors fixed to the Fc part of IgG1. As it is not a mAb, it may also be less immunogenic. This may explain the reported lack of ADAb to ETN [18] even in RA patients followed up for five years [120]. Despite being a mAb, GOL had low levels of ADAb – 2.1% in GO-FORWARD [44] and 3% in GO-AFTER [47].

ACCOMPANY was a multicenter, open-label study consisting of a short-term treatment period (to day 113) and a LTE period to assess the immunogenicity, safety, and efficacy of SC ABA with or without concomitant MTX [121]. No patient who received ABA + MTX (n = 50) or ABA alone (n = 45) had ADAb detectable by ELISA at day 113 [121].

Similarly, ADAb to SC TCZ were seen only at very low levels in the SUMMACTA trial (0.8%) [14]. This finding has been noted in all Phase III TCZ clinical trials [122]. The inhibitory effect of IL-6 blockade on B-cell activity may be at least partly responsible for this.

Maintenance of a constant trough level of the biologic agent may facilitate optimal disease control and prevention of ADAb development. In contrast, intermittent appearance of an antigen (in this case, a bDMARD) may promote an immune response manifested as an ADAb [111]. Given the technical difficulty with ADAb measurement and the variability between different assays, a serum drug trough concentration may have the most clinical utility.

Primary failure to a bDMARD in the setting of adequate medication adherence [123] suggests the choice of therapeutic target may not be appropriate and an alternative bDMARD class may need to be tried (Figure 1). Secondary failure with adequate medication adherence and a low serum trough level may indicate the presence of ADAb, which may be detected with one of the techniques discussed above. While this may be overcome by increasing the bDMARD dose, depending on the local regulatory environment, this may not be possible. Data from the British Society of Rheumatology Biologics Registry (BSRBR) has shown that RA patients switched to a second TNFi following lack of response to a first TNFi have high rates of drug continuation [124]. These findings suggest that loss of efficacy may be due to immunogenicity to that TNFi and therefore switching to a different bDMARD in the same therapeutic class is a rational option. As MTX appeared to inhibit ADAb development, it seems wise to use this in combination with IFX [117] and ADL [115, 119]. As ETN [18, 120], GOL [7, 38] and the non-TNFi bDMARDS [14, 121, 122] appear less likely to develop ADAb, MTX co-administration may not be required if disease control is adequate with bDMARD monotherapy.

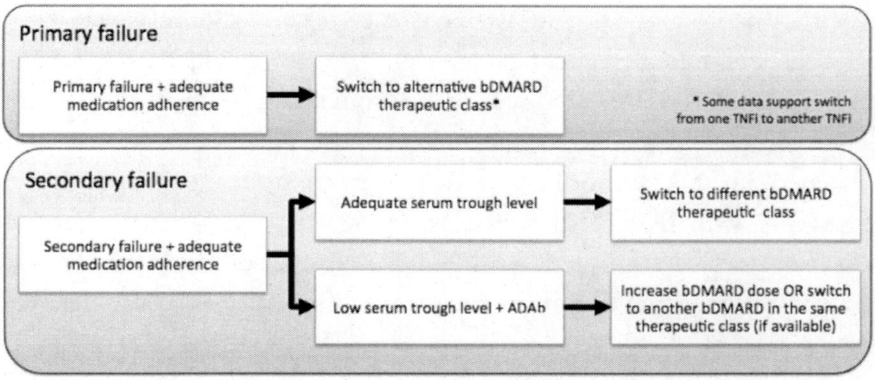


Figure 1. Possible therapeutic strategies using serum trough bDMARD levels and anti-drug neutralising antibody (ADAb) assay.

## A Practical Approach to Drug Choice

The increasing number and availability of bDMARDS and tsDMARDS means it can be difficult to know which agent to use. This section outlines a practical approach to bDMARD choice. As most bDMARDS and tsDMARDS have similar efficacy because they all act on a common pathway, namely the pro-inflammatory cascade, drug choice is usually determined by physician familiarity with the drug, national regulatory prescribing guidelines, side effect profile and route/frequency of administration.

As TNFi's were the first class of targeted therapy available, most Rheumatologists use these as first-line bDMARDS. Within this drug class, the 4-weekly administration of GOL may improve drug adherence [49] and may be preferred by patients who dislike parenteral drugs. The weekly administration of ETN may be helpful in those at high risk of infection as cessation allows rapid drug clearance; ETN is also associated with a lower risk of Mycobacterial infection [24, 25]. The fortnightly administration of

ADL and CZP provides a compromise between the frequency of GOL (every 4 weeks) and ETN (weekly). The established track record of ADL is reassuring – although it appears to have a higher risk of ADAb [108]. While CZP is usually given at a maintenance dose of 200 mg every two weeks, the well-tolerated loading dose of 400 mg at week 0, 2 and 4 means double doses of 200 mg x 2 can be given from time-to-time, especially in heavier patients when RA flares. Generally, TNFi's should be co-administered with MTX for better efficacy and to lower the risk of ADAb – especially with IFX [117] and ADL [115, 119]. Primary failure of a TNFi does not necessarily mean a bDMARD from a different therapeutic class should be an automatic choice as a second TNFi can often be effective [2].

It would also be reasonable to use TCZ as a first-line bDMARD, particularly in the setting of MTX intolerance. Tocilizumab appears superior to ADL as monotherapy [57]. The lack of ADAb, possibly due to the inhibitory effect of IL-6 blockade on B-lymphocyte function, is reassuring [122]. However, TCZ is probably best avoided in the setting of previous diverticulitis [56]. The lack of association with NMSC means TCZ is preferable to a TNFi in the setting of skin cancer.

Co-stimulation blockade with ABA appears to have a lower risk of infection than TNFi [70]. It may be the bDMARD of choice in those at high risk of infection. The weekly administration allows rapid drug clearance if infection occurs.

In most countries, RTX is only licensed for use in the setting of TNFi failure. The two infusions at week 0 and 2, which only need to be given every six months, are convenient. While the persistent peripheral blood B-lymphocyte depletion is daunting, it appears well tolerated [81]. However, the duration of B-lymphocyte depletion means vaccination should occur prior to the first RTX infusion [125]. Its long history of use for the treatment of lymphoma means most Rheumatologists are comfortable using RTX in patients with a history of malignancy.

The recent availability of TFN as the first oral small molecule inhibitor is a major advance and heralds another new phase in RA treatment. It is particularly useful for those who have difficulty with injections as all the other bDMARDS are administered parenterally. The increased risk of shingles, especially in Asians [91], means administration of the live shingles vaccine should be considered prior to commencement of TFN [125].

## Summary

The increasing range of bDMARDS and tsDMARDS has revolutionised the treatment of RA and will also be beneficial for management of other forms of inflammatory arthritis and immune-mediated diseases. As most bDMARDS and tsDMARDS have similar efficacy because they all act on the pro-inflammatory cascade, drug choice is usually determined by physician familiarity with the drug, national regulatory prescribing guidelines, side effect profile and route/frequency of administration. It is hoped that ongoing efforts to identify prognostic biomarkers to assist in choice of DMARD will be of clinical utility. The development of ADAb may be responsible for secondary failure to a bDMARD – especially in the case of ADL and IFX. The use of MTX may be protective against this. Although more trials involving biosilimars are required, it is hoped their increasing availability will lower the cost of treating patients and increase access to optimal bDMARD therapy for patients with inflammatory arthritis.

# References

[1] Singh JA, Saag KG, Bridges SL, Jr., et al. 2015 American College of Rheumatology Guideline for the Treatment of Rheumatoid Arthritis. *Arthritis Rheumatol*. 2016;68:1-26.

[2] Smolen JS, Aletaha D, McInnes IB. Rheumatoid arthritis. *Lancet*. 2016;388:2023-38.

[3] Burmester GR, Pope JE. Novel treatment strategies in rheumatoid arthritis. *Lancet*. 2017;389:2338-48.

[4] Bansback N, Phibbs CS, Sun H, et al. Triple Therapy Versus Biologic Therapy for Active Rheumatoid Arthritis: A Cost-Effectiveness Analysis. *Ann Intern Med.* 2017;167:8-16.

[5] Genovese MC, McKay JD, Nasonov EL, et al. Interleukin-6 receptor inhibition with tocilizumab reduces disease activity in rheumatoid arthritis with inadequate response to disease-modifying antirheumatic drugs: the tocilizumab in combination with traditional disease-modifying antirheumatic drug therapy study. *Arthritis Rheum*. 2008;58:2968-80.

[6] Yoo DH, Hrycaj P, Miranda P, et al. A randomised, double-blind, parallel-group study to demonstrate equivalence in efficacy and safety of CT-P13 compared with innovator infliximab when coadministered with methotrexate in patients with active rheumatoid arthritis: the PLANETRA study. *Ann Rheum Dis*. 2013;72:1613-20.

[7] Keystone E, Heijde D, Mason D, Jr., et al. Certolizumab pegol plus methotrexate is significantly more effective than placebo plus methotrexate in active rheumatoid arthritis: findings of a fifty-two-week, phase III, multicenter, randomized, double-blind, placebo-controlled, parallel-group study. *Arthritis Rheum*. 2008;58:3319-29.

[8] Schiff M, Pritchard C, Huffstutter JE, et al. The 6-month safety and efficacy of abatacept in patients with rheumatoid arthritis who underwent a washout after anti-tumour necrosis factor therapy or were directly switched to abatacept: the ARRIVE trial. *Ann Rheum Dis*. 2009;68:1708-14.

[9] Fleischmann R, Kremer J, Cush J, et al. Placebo-controlled trial of tofacitinib monotherapy in rheumatoid arthritis. *N Engl J Med.* 2012;367:495-507.

[10] Emery P, Bingham CO, 3rd, Burmester GR, et al. Certolizumab pegol in combination with dose-optimised methotrexate in DMARD-naive patients with early, active rheumatoid arthritis with poor prognostic factors: 1-year results from C-EARLY, a randomised, double-blind, placebo-controlled phase III study. *Ann Rheum Dis*. 2017;76:96-104.

[11] Breedveld FC, Weisman MH, Kavanaugh AF, et al. The PREMIER study: A multicenter, randomized, double-blind clinical trial of combination therapy with adalimumab plus methotrexate versus methotrexate alone or adalimumab alone in patients with early, aggressive rheumatoid arthritis who had not had previous methotrexate treatment. *Arthritis Rheum*. 2006;54:26-37.

[12] Kavanaugh A, Fleischmann RM, Emery P, et al. Clinical, functional and radiographic consequences of achieving stable low disease activity and remission with adalimumab plus methotrexate or methotrexate alone in early rheumatoid arthritis: 26-week results from the randomised, controlled OPTIMA study. *Ann Rheum Dis*. 2013;72:64-71.

[13] Weinblatt ME, Schiff M, Valente R, et al. Head-to-head comparison of subcutaneous abatacept versus adalimumab for rheumatoid arthritis: findings of a phase IIIb, multinational, prospective, randomized study. *Arthritis Rheum*. 2013;65:28-38.

[14] Burmester GR, Rubbert-Roth A, Cantagrel A, et al. A randomised, double-blind, parallel-group study of the safety and efficacy of subcutaneous tocilizumab versus intravenous tocilizumab in combination with traditional disease-modifying antirheumatic drugs in patients with moderate to severe rheumatoid arthritis (SUMMACTA study). *Ann Rheum Dis*. 2014;73:69-74.

[15] Emery P, Burmester GR, Bykerk VP, et al. Evaluating drug-free remission with abatacept in early rheumatoid arthritis: results from the phase 3b, multicentre, randomised, active-controlled AVERT study of 24 months, with a 12-month, double-blind treatment period. *Ann Rheum Dis*. 2015;74:19-26.

[16] Kaine J, Gladstein G, Strusberg I, et al. Evaluation of abatacept administered subcutaneously in adults with active rheumatoid arthritis: impact of withdrawal and reintroduction on immunogenicity, efficacy and safety (phase IIIb ALLOW study). *Ann Rheum Dis*. 2012;71:38-44.

[17] Mohler KM, Torrance DS, Smith CA, et al. Soluble tumor necrosis factor (TNF) receptors are effective therapeutic agents in lethal

endotoxemia and function simultaneously as both TNF carriers and TNF antagonists. *J Immunol.* 1993;151:1548-61.

[18] Weinblatt ME, Kremer JM, Bankhurst AD, et al. A trial of etanercept, a recombinant tumor necrosis factor receptor:Fc fusion protein, in patients with rheumatoid arthritis receiving methotrexate. *N Engl J Med.* 1999;340:253-9.

[19] Klareskog L, van der Heijde D, de Jager JP, et al. Therapeutic effect of the combination of etanercept and methotrexate compared with each treatment alone in patients with rheumatoid arthritis: double-blind randomised controlled trial. *Lancet.* 2004;363:675-81.

[20] Emery P, Breedveld FC, Hall S, et al. Comparison of methotrexate monotherapy with a combination of methotrexate and etanercept in active, early, moderate to severe rheumatoid arthritis (COMET): a randomised, double-blind, parallel treatment trial. *Lancet.* 2008;372:375-82.

[21] Emery P, Breedveld F, van der Heijde D, et al. Two-year clinical and radiographic results with combination etanercept-methotrexate therapy versus monotherapy in early rheumatoid arthritis: a two-year, double-blind, randomized study. *Arthritis Rheum.* 2010;62:674-82.

[22] Combe B, Codreanu C, Fiocco U, et al. Etanercept and sulfasalazine, alone and combined, in patients with active rheumatoid arthritis despite receiving sulfasalazine: a double-blind comparison. *Ann Rheum Dis.* 2006;65:1357-62.

[23] Smolen JS, Nash P, Durez P, et al. Maintenance, reduction, or withdrawal of etanercept after treatment with etanercept and methotrexate in patients with moderate rheumatoid arthritis (PRESERVE): a randomised controlled trial. *Lancet.* 2013;381:918-29.

[24] Winthrop KL, Siegel JN, Jereb J, Taylor Z, Iademarco MF. Tuberculosis associated with therapy against tumor necrosis factor alpha. *Arthritis Rheum.* 2005;52:2968-74.

[25] Cantini F, Niccoli L, Goletti D. Adalimumab, etanercept, infliximab, and the risk of tuberculosis: data from clinical trials,

national registries, and postmarketing surveillance. *J Rheumatol Suppl*. 2014;91:47-55.

[26] Sandborn WJ, Hanauer SB, Katz S, et al. Etanercept for active Crohn's disease: a randomized, double-blind, placebo-controlled trial. *Gastroenterology*. 2001;121:1088-94.

[27] Salfeld. J, Kaymakcalan. Z, Tracey. D, Roberts. A, R. K. Generation of fully human anti-TNF antibody D2E7 [abstract]. *Arthritis Rheum*. 1998;41:S57.

[28] Keystone EC, Kavanaugh AF, Sharp JT, et al. Radiographic, clinical, and functional outcomes of treatment with adalimumab (a human anti-tumor necrosis factor monoclonal antibody) in patients with active rheumatoid arthritis receiving concomitant methotrexate therapy: a randomized, placebo-controlled, 52-week trial. *Arthritis Rheum*. 2004;50:1400-11.

[29] Keystone EC, van der Heijde D, Kavanaugh A, et al. Clinical, functional, and radiographic benefits of longterm adalimumab plus methotrexate: final 10-year data in longstanding rheumatoid arthritis. *J Rheumatol*. 2013;40:1487-97.

[30] Keystone EC, Breedveld FC, van der Heijde D, et al. Longterm effect of delaying combination therapy with tumor necrosis factor inhibitor in patients with aggressive early rheumatoid arthritis: 10-year efficacy and safety of adalimumab from the randomized controlled PREMIER trial with open-label extension. *J Rheumatol*. 2014;41:5-14.

[31] Smolen JS, Emery P, Fleischmann R, et al. Adjustment of therapy in rheumatoid arthritis on the basis of achievement of stable low disease activity with adalimumab plus methotrexate or methotrexate alone: the randomised controlled OPTIMA trial. *Lancet*. 2014;383:321-32.

[32] Knight DM, Trinh H, Le J, et al. Construction and initial characterization of a mouse-human chimeric anti-TNF antibody. *Mol Immunol*. 1993;30:1443-53.

[33] Maini R, St Clair EW, Breedveld F, et al. Infliximab (chimeric anti-tumour necrosis factor alpha monoclonal antibody) versus placebo

in rheumatoid arthritis patients receiving concomitant methotrexate: a randomised phase III trial. ATTRACT Study Group. *Lancet.* 1999;354:1932-9.

[34] Maini RN, Breedveld FC, Kalden JR, et al. Sustained improvement over two years in physical function, structural damage, and signs and symptoms among patients with rheumatoid arthritis treated with infliximab and methotrexate. *Arthritis Rheum*. 2004;50:1051-65.

[35] St Clair EW, van der Heijde DM, Smolen JS, et al. Combination of infliximab and methotrexate therapy for early rheumatoid arthritis: a randomized, controlled trial. *Arthritis Rheum*. 2004;50:3432-43.

[36] Westhovens R, Yocum D, Han J, et al. The safety of infliximab, combined with background treatments, among patients with rheumatoid arthritis and various comorbidities: a large, randomized, placebo-controlled trial. *Arthritis Rheum*. 2006;54:1075-86.

[37] Nesbitt A, Fossati G, Bergin M, et al. Mechanism of action of certolizumab pegol (CDP870): in vitro comparison with other anti-tumor necrosis factor alpha agents. *Inflamm Bowel Dis*. 2007;13:1323-32.

[38] Smolen J, Landewe RB, Mease P, et al. Efficacy and safety of certolizumab pegol plus methotrexate in active rheumatoid arthritis: the RAPID 2 study. A randomised controlled trial. *Ann Rheum Dis*. 2009;68:797-804.

[39] Fleischmann R, Vencovsky J, van Vollenhoven RF, et al. Efficacy and safety of certolizumab pegol monotherapy every 4 weeks in patients with rheumatoid arthritis failing previous disease-modifying antirheumatic therapy: the FAST4WARD study. *Ann Rheum Dis*. 2009;68:805-11.

[40] Choy E, McKenna F, Vencovsky J, et al. Certolizumab pegol plus MTX administered every 4 weeks is effective in patients with RA who are partial responders to MTX. *Rheumatology* (Oxford). 2012;51:1226-34.

[41] Smolen JS, Burmester GR, Combe B, et al. Head-to-head comparison of certolizumab pegol versus adalimumab in

rheumatoid arthritis: 2-year efficacy and safety results from the randomised EXXELERATE study. *Lancet*. 2016;388:2763-74.

[42] Clowse ME, Forger F, Hwang C, et al. Minimal to no transfer of certolizumab pegol into breast milk: results from CRADLE, a prospective, postmarketing, multicentre, pharmacokinetic study. *Ann Rheum Dis*. 2017;76:1890-6.

[43] Fishwild DM, O'Donnell SL, Bengoechea T, et al. High-avidity human IgG kappa monoclonal antibodies from a novel strain of minilocus transgenic mice. *Nat Biotechnol*. 1996;14:845-51.

[44] Keystone EC, Genovese MC, Klareskog L, et al. Golimumab, a human antibody to tumour necrosis factor {alpha} given by monthly subcutaneous injections, in active rheumatoid arthritis despite methotrexate therapy: the GO-FORWARD Study. *Ann Rheum Dis*. 2009;68:789-96.

[45] Keystone E, Genovese MC, Klareskog L, et al. Golimumab in patients with active rheumatoid arthritis despite methotrexate therapy: 52-week results of the GO-FORWARD study. *Ann Rheum Dis*. 2010;69:1129-35.

[46] Keystone EC, Genovese MC, Hall S, et al. Safety and Efficacy of Subcutaneous Golimumab in Patients with Active Rheumatoid Arthritis despite Methotrexate Therapy: Final 5-year Results of the GO-FORWARD Trial. *J Rheumatol*. 2016;43:298-306.

[47] Smolen JS, Kay J, Doyle MK, et al. Golimumab in patients with active rheumatoid arthritis after treatment with tumour necrosis factor alpha inhibitors (GO-AFTER study): a multicentre, randomised, double-blind, placebo-controlled, phase III trial. *Lancet*. 2009;374:210-21.

[48] Smolen JS, Kay J, Doyle M, et al. Golimumab in patients with active rheumatoid arthritis after treatment with tumor necrosis factor alpha inhibitors: findings with up to five years of treatment in the multicenter, randomized, double-blind, placebo-controlled, phase 3 GO-AFTER study. *Arthritis Res Ther*. 2015;17:14.

[49] Bhoi P, Bessette L, Bell MJ, Tkaczyk C, Nantel F, Maslova K. Adherence and dosing interval of subcutaneous antitumour necrosis

factor biologics among patients with inflammatory arthritis: analysis from a Canadian administrative database. *BMJ Open*. 2017;7:e015872.

[50] Wong PK, Campbell IK, Egan PJ, Ernst M, Wicks IP. The role of the interleukin-6 family of cytokines in inflammatory arthritis and bone turnover. *Arthritis Rheum*. 2003;48:1177-89.

[51] Wong PK, Quinn JM, Sims NA, van Nieuwenhuijze A, Campbell IK, Wicks IP. Interleukin-6 modulates production of T lymphocyte-derived cytokines in antigen-induced arthritis and drives inflammation-induced osteoclastogenesis. *Arthritis Rheum*. 2006;54:158-68.

[52] Smolen JS, Beaulieu A, Rubbert-Roth A, et al. Effect of interleukin-6 receptor inhibition with tocilizumab in patients with rheumatoid arthritis (OPTION study): a double-blind, placebo-controlled, randomised trial. *Lancet*. 2008;371:987-97.

[53] Wright HL, Cross AL, Edwards SW, Moots RJ. Effects of IL-6 and IL-6 blockade on neutrophil function in vitro and in vivo. *Rheumatology* (Oxford). 2014;53:1321-31.

[54] Kremer JM, Blanco R, Brzosko M, et al. Tocilizumab inhibits structural joint damage in rheumatoid arthritis patients with inadequate responses to methotrexate: results from the double-blind treatment phase of a randomized placebo-controlled trial of tocilizumab safety and prevention of structural joint damage at one year. *Arthritis Rheum*. 2011;63:609-21.

[55] Jones G, Sebba A, Gu J, et al. Comparison of tocilizumab monotherapy versus methotrexate monotherapy in patients with moderate to severe rheumatoid arthritis: the AMBITION study. *Ann Rheum Dis*. 2010;69:88-96.

[56] Emery P, Keystone E, Tony HP, et al. IL-6 receptor inhibition with tocilizumab improves treatment outcomes in patients with rheumatoid arthritis refractory to anti-tumour necrosis factor biologicals: results from a 24-week multicentre randomised placebo-controlled trial. *Ann Rheum Dis*. 2008;67:1516-23.

[57] Gabay C, Emery P, van Vollenhoven R, et al. Tocilizumab monotherapy versus adalimumab monotherapy for treatment of rheumatoid arthritis (ADACTA): a randomised, double-blind, controlled phase 4 trial. *Lancet*. 2013;381:1541-50.

[58] Dougados M, Kissel K, Conaghan PG, et al. Clinical, radiographic and immunogenic effects after 1 year of tocilizumab-based treatment strategies in rheumatoid arthritis: the ACT-RAY study. *Ann Rheum Dis*. 2014;73:803-9.

[59] Souto A, Salgado E, Maneiro JR, Mera A, Carmona L, Gomez-Reino JJ. Lipid profile changes in patients with chronic inflammatory arthritis treated with biologic agents and tofacitinib in randomized clinical trials: a systematic review and meta-analysis. *Arthritis Rheumatol*. 2015;67:117-27.

[60] Rao VU, Pavlov A, Klearman M, et al. An evaluation of risk factors for major adverse cardiovascular events during tocilizumab therapy. *Arthritis Rheumatol*. 2015;67:372-80.

[61] Andrews NC. Anemia of inflammation: the cytokine-hepcidin link. *J Clin Invest*. 2004;113:1251-3.

[62] Genovese MC, Fleischmann R, Kivitz AJ, et al. Sarilumab Plus Methotrexate in Patients With Active Rheumatoid Arthritis and Inadequate Response to Methotrexate: Results of a Phase III Study. *Arthritis Rheumatol*. 2015;67:1424-37.

[63] Burmester GR, Lin Y, Patel R, et al. Efficacy and safety of sarilumab monotherapy versus adalimumab monotherapy for the treatment of patients with active rheumatoid arthritis (MONARCH): a randomised, double-blind, parallel-group phase III trial. *Ann Rheum Dis*. 2017;76:840-7.

[64] Smolen JS, Weinblatt ME, Sheng S, Zhuang Y, Hsu B. Sirukumab, a human anti-interleukin-6 monoclonal antibody: a randomised, 2-part (proof-of-concept and dose-finding), phase II study in patients with active rheumatoid arthritis despite methotrexate therapy. *Ann Rheum Dis*. 2014;73:1616-25.

[65] Moreland LW, Alten R, Van den Bosch F, et al. Costimulatory blockade in patients with rheumatoid arthritis: a pilot, dose-finding,

double-blind, placebo-controlled clinical trial evaluating CTLA-4Ig and LEA29Y eighty-five days after the first infusion. *Arthritis Rheum*. 2002;46:1470-9.

[66] Kremer JM, Genant HK, Moreland LW, et al. Effects of abatacept in patients with methotrexate-resistant active rheumatoid arthritis: a randomized trial. *Ann Intern Med*. 2006;144:865-76.

[67] Genovese MC, Becker JC, Schiff M, et al. Abatacept for rheumatoid arthritis refractory to tumor necrosis factor alpha inhibition. *N Engl J Med*. 2005;353:1114-23.

[68] Westhovens R, Robles M, Ximenes AC, et al. Clinical efficacy and safety of abatacept in methotrexate-naive patients with early rheumatoid arthritis and poor prognostic factors. *Ann Rheum Dis*. 2009;68:1870-7.

[69] Emery P, Durez P, Dougados M, et al. Impact of T-cell costimulation modulation in patients with undifferentiated inflammatory arthritis or very early rheumatoid arthritis: a clinical and imaging study of abatacept (the ADJUST trial). *Ann Rheum Dis*. 2010;69:510-6.

[70] Schiff M, Keiserman M, Codding C, et al. Efficacy and safety of abatacept or infliximab vs placebo in ATTEST: a phase III, multicentre, randomised, double-blind, placebo-controlled study in patients with rheumatoid arthritis and an inadequate response to methotrexate. *Ann Rheum Dis*. 2008;67:1096-103.

[71] Hodi FS, O'Day SJ, McDermott DF, et al. Improved survival with ipilimumab in patients with metastatic melanoma. *N Engl J Med*. 2010;363:711-23.

[72] Maneiro JR, Souto A, Gomez-Reino JJ. Risks of malignancies related to tofacitinib and biological drugs in rheumatoid arthritis: Systematic review, meta-analysis, and network meta-analysis. *Semin Arthritis Rheum*. 2017;47:149-56.

[73] Simon TA, Smitten AL, Franklin J, et al. Malignancies in the rheumatoid arthritis abatacept clinical development programme: an epidemiological assessment. *Ann Rheum Dis*. 2009;68:1819-26.

[74] Scott FI, Mamtani R, Brensinger CM, et al. Risk of Nonmelanoma Skin Cancer Associated With the Use of Immunosuppressant and Biologic Agents in Patients With a History of Autoimmune Disease and Nonmelanoma Skin Cancer. *JAMA Dermatol*. 2016;152:164-72.

[75] Anderson DR, Grillo-Lopez A, Varns C, Chambers KS, Hanna N. Targeted anti-cancer therapy using rituximab, a chimaeric anti-CD20 antibody (IDEC-C2B8) in the treatment of non-Hodgkin's B-cell lymphoma. *Biochem Soc Trans*. 1997;25:705-8.

[76] Clynes RA, Towers TL, Presta LG, Ravetch JV. Inhibitory Fc receptors modulate in vivo cytotoxicity against tumor targets. *Nat Med*. 2000;6:443-6.

[77] Reff ME, Carner K, Chambers KS, et al. Depletion of B cells in vivo by a chimeric mouse human monoclonal antibody to CD20. *Blood*. 1994;83:435-45.

[78] Tak PP, Rigby WF, Rubbert-Roth A, et al. Inhibition of joint damage and improved clinical outcomes with rituximab plus methotrexate in early active rheumatoid arthritis: the IMAGE trial. *Ann Rheum Dis*. 2011;70:39-46.

[79] Emery P, Deodhar A, Rigby WF, et al. Efficacy and safety of different doses and retreatment of rituximab: a randomised, placebo-controlled trial in patients who are biological naive with active rheumatoid arthritis and an inadequate response to methotrexate (Study Evaluating Rituximab's Efficacy in MTX iNadequate rEsponders (SERENE)). *Ann Rheum Dis*. 2010;69:1629-35.

[80] Emery P, Fleischmann R, Filipowicz-Sosnowska A, et al. The efficacy and safety of rituximab in patients with active rheumatoid arthritis despite methotrexate treatment: results of a phase IIB randomized, double-blind, placebo-controlled, dose-ranging trial. *Arthritis Rheum*. 2006;54:1390-400.

[81] Cohen SB, Emery P, Greenwald MW, et al. Rituximab for rheumatoid arthritis refractory to anti-tumor necrosis factor therapy: Results of a multicenter, randomized, double-blind, placebo-

controlled, phase III trial evaluating primary efficacy and safety at twenty-four weeks. *Arthritis Rheum.* 2006;54:2793-806.

[82] Meyer DM, Jesson MI, Li X, et al. Anti-inflammatory activity and neutrophil reductions mediated by the JAK1/JAK3 inhibitor, CP-690,550, in rat adjuvant-induced arthritis. *J Inflamm (Lond).* 2010;7:41.

[83] Flanagan ME, Blumenkopf TA, Brissette WH, et al. Discovery of CP-690,550: a potent and selective Janus kinase (JAK) inhibitor for the treatment of autoimmune diseases and organ transplant rejection. *J Med Chem.* 2010;53:8468-84.

[84] Clark JD, Flanagan ME, Telliez JB. Discovery and development of Janus kinase (JAK) inhibitors for inflammatory diseases. *J Med Chem.* 2014;57:5023-38.

[85] Lee EB, Fleischmann R, Hall S, et al. Tofacitinib versus methotrexate in rheumatoid arthritis. *N Engl J Med.* 2014;370:2377-86.

[86] Bruynesteyn K, van der Heijde D, Boers M, et al. Determination of the minimal clinically important difference in rheumatoid arthritis joint damage of the Sharp/van der Heijde and Larsen/Scott scoring methods by clinical experts and comparison with the smallest detectable difference. *Arthritis Rheum.* 2002;46:913-20.

[87] Kremer J, Li ZG, Hall S, et al. Tofacitinib in combination with nonbiologic disease-modifying antirheumatic drugs in patients with active rheumatoid arthritis: a randomized trial. *Ann Intern Med.* 2013;159:253-61.

[88] van Vollenhoven RF, Fleischmann R, Cohen S, et al. Tofacitinib or adalimumab versus placebo in rheumatoid arthritis. *N Engl J Med.* 2012;367:508-19.

[89] Fleischmann R, Mysler E, Hall S, et al. Efficacy and safety of tofacitinib monotherapy, tofacitinib with methotrexate, and adalimumab with methotrexate in patients with rheumatoid arthritis (ORAL Strategy): a phase 3b/4, double-blind, head-to-head, randomised controlled trial. *Lancet.* 2017;390:457-68.

[90] Burmester GR, Blanco R, Charles-Schoeman C, et al. Tofacitinib (CP-690,550) in combination with methotrexate in patients with active rheumatoid arthritis with an inadequate response to tumour necrosis factor inhibitors: a randomised phase 3 trial. *Lancet*. 2013;381:451-60.

[91] Winthrop KL, Curtis JR, Lindsey S, et al. Herpes Zoster and Tofacitinib: Clinical Outcomes and the Risk of Concomitant Therapy. *Arthritis Rheumatol*. 2017;69:1960-8.

[92] Dougados M, van der Heijde D, Chen YC, et al. Baricitinib in patients with inadequate response or intolerance to conventional synthetic DMARDs: results from the RA-BUILD study. *Ann Rheum Dis*. 2017;76:88-95.

[93] Genovese MC, Kremer J, Zamani O, et al. Baricitinib in Patients with Refractory Rheumatoid Arthritis. *N Engl J Med*. 2016;374:1243-52.

[94] Taylor PC, Keystone EC, van der Heijde D, et al. Baricitinib versus Placebo or Adalimumab in Rheumatoid Arthritis. *N Engl J Med*. 2017;376:652-62.

[95] Schellekens H, Lietzan E, Faccin F, Venema J. Biosimilar monoclonal antibodies: the scientific basis for extrapolation. *Expert Opin Biol Ther*. 2015;15:1633-46.

[96] Ebbers HC, Crow SA, Vulto AG, Schellekens H. Interchangeability, immunogenicity and biosimilars. *Nat Biotechnol*. 2012;30:1186-90.

[97] Weise M, Kurki P, Wolff-Holz E, Bielsky MC, Schneider CK. Biosimilars: the science of extrapolation. *Blood*. 2014;124:3191-6.

[98] American College of Rheumatology. *Position Statement: Biosimilars* https://www.rheumatology.org/Portals/0/Files/Biosimilars-Position-Statement.pdf 2016 [Accessed: 31 October 2017].

[99] Australian Rheumatology Association. *ARA Position on the Introduction of Biosimilars for the Treatment of Rheumatic Diseases*: https://rheumatology.org.au/downloads/ARApositionstatementbiosimilarsNov16final.pdf 2016 [Accessed: 31 October 2017].

[100] Declerck PJ. Biologicals and biosimilars: a review of the science and its implications. *Generics and Biosimilars Initiative Journal*. 2012;1:13-6.

[101] Jorgensen KK, Olsen IC, Goll GL, et al. Switching from originator infliximab to biosimilar CT-P13 compared with maintained treatment with originator infliximab (NOR-SWITCH): a 52-week, randomised, double-blind, non-inferiority trial. *Lancet*. 2017;389:2304-16.

[102] Glintborg B, Sorensen IJ, Loft AG, et al. A nationwide non-medical switch from originator infliximab to biosimilar CT-P13 in 802 patients with inflammatory arthritis: 1-year clinical outcomes from the DANBIO registry. *Ann Rheum Dis*. 2017;76:1426-31.

[103] Smolen JS, Choe JY, Prodanovic N, et al. Safety, immunogenicity and efficacy after switching from reference infliximab to biosimilar SB2 compared with continuing reference infliximab and SB2 in patients with rheumatoid arthritis: results of a randomised, double-blind, phase III transition study. *Ann Rheum Dis*. 2017;77:234-40.

[104] Emery P, Vencovsky J, Sylwestrzak A, et al. A phase III randomised, double-blind, parallel-group study comparing SB4 with etanercept reference product in patients with active rheumatoid arthritis despite methotrexate therapy. *Ann Rheum Dis*. 2017;76:51-7.

[105] Emery P, Vencovsky J, Sylwestrzak A, et al. Long-term efficacy and safety in patients with rheumatoid arthritis continuing on SB4 or switching from reference etanercept to SB4. *Ann Rheum Dis*. 2017; in press

[106] Bae SC, Kim J, Choe JY, et al. A phase III, multicentre, randomised, double-blind, active-controlled, parallel-group trial comparing safety and efficacy of HD203, with innovator etanercept, in combination with methotrexate, in patients with rheumatoid arthritis: the HERA study. *Ann Rheum Dis*. 2017;76:65-71.

[107] Kay J, Schoels MM, Dorner T, et al. Consensus-based recommendations for the use of biosimilars to treat rheumatological diseases. *Ann Rheum Dis*. 2017;77;165-74.

[108] Vincent FB, Morand EF, Murphy K, Mackay F, Mariette X, Marcelli C. Antidrug antibodies (ADAb) to tumour necrosis factor (TNF)-specific neutralising agents in chronic inflammatory diseases: a real issue, a clinical perspective. *Ann Rheum Dis*. 2013;72:165-78.

[109] van der Laken CJ, Voskuyl AE, Roos JC, et al. Imaging and serum analysis of immune complex formation of radiolabelled infliximab and anti-infliximab in responders and non-responders to therapy for rheumatoid arthritis. *Ann Rheum Dis*. 2007;66:253-6.

[110] van Schouwenburg PA, van de Stadt LA, de Jong RN, et al. Adalimumab elicits a restricted anti-idiotypic antibody response in autoimmune patients resulting in functional neutralisation. *Ann Rheum Dis*. 2013;72:104-9.

[111] Schaeverbeke T, Truchetet ME, Kostine M, Barnetche T, Bannwarth B, Richez C. Immunogenicity of biologic agents in rheumatoid arthritis patients: lessons for clinical practice. *Rheumatology (Oxford)*. 2016;55:210-20.

[112] van Schouwenburg PA, Krieckaert CL, Rispens T, Aarden L, Wolbink GJ, Wouters D. Long-term measurement of anti-adalimumab using pH-shift-anti-idiotype antigen binding test shows predictive value and transient antibody formation. *Ann Rheum Dis*. 2013;72:1680-6.

[113] Bartelds GM, Krieckaert CL, Nurmohamed MT, et al. Development of antidrug antibodies against adalimumab and association with disease activity and treatment failure during long-term follow-up. *JAMA*. 2011;305:1460-8.

[114] Krieckaert CL, Jamnitski A, Nurmohamed MT, Kostense PJ, Boers M, Wolbink G. Comparison of long-term clinical outcome with etanercept treatment and adalimumab treatment of rheumatoid arthritis with respect to immunogenicity. *Arthritis Rheum*. 2012;64:3850-5.

[115] Krieckaert CL, Nurmohamed MT, Wolbink GJ. Methotrexate reduces immunogenicity in adalimumab treated rheumatoid arthritis

patients in a dose dependent manner. *Ann Rheum Dis.* 2012;71:1914-5.

[116] Bendtzen K, Geborek P, Svenson M, Larsson L, Kapetanovic MC, Saxne T. Individualized monitoring of drug bioavailability and immunogenicity in rheumatoid arthritis patients treated with the tumor necrosis factor alpha inhibitor infliximab. *Arthritis Rheum.* 2006;54:3782-9.

[117] Maini RN, Breedveld FC, Kalden JR, et al. Therapeutic efficacy of multiple intravenous infusions of anti-tumor necrosis factor alpha monoclonal antibody combined with low-dose weekly methotrexate in rheumatoid arthritis. *Arthritis Rheum.* 1998;41:1552-63.

[118] Radstake TR, Svenson M, Eijsbouts AM, et al. Formation of antibodies against infliximab and adalimumab strongly correlates with functional drug levels and clinical responses in rheumatoid arthritis. *Ann Rheum Dis.* 2009;68:1739-45.

[119] Garces S, Demengeot J, Benito-Garcia E. The immunogenicity of anti-TNF therapy in immune-mediated inflammatory diseases: a systematic review of the literature with a meta-analysis. *Ann Rheum Dis.* 2013;72:1947-55.

[120] Klareskog L, Gaubitz M, Rodriguez-Valverde V, et al. Assessment of long-term safety and efficacy of etanercept in a 5-year extension study in patients with rheumatoid arthritis. *Clin Exp Rheumatol.* 2011;29:238-47.

[121] Nash P, Nayiager S, Genovese MC, et al. Immunogenicity, safety, and efficacy of abatacept administered subcutaneously with or without background methotrexate in patients with rheumatoid arthritis: results from a phase III, international, multicenter, parallel-arm, open-label study. *Arthritis Care Res (Hoboken).* 2013;65:718-28.

[122] Stubenrauch K, Wessels U, Birnboeck H, Ramirez F, Jahreis A, Schleypen J. Subset analysis of patients experiencing clinical events of a potentially immunogenic nature in the pivotal clinical trials of tocilizumab for rheumatoid arthritis: Evaluation of an antidrug

antibody ELISA using clinical adverse event-driven immunogenicity testing. *Clin Ther*. 2010;32:1597-609.

[123] Wong PK. Medication adherence in patients with rheumatoid arthritis: why do patients not take what we prescribe? *Rheumatol Int*. 2016;36:1535-42.

[124] Hyrich KL, Lunt M, Watson KD, Symmons DP, Silman AJ, British Society for Rheumatology Biologics R. Outcomes after switching from one anti-tumor necrosis factor alpha agent to a second anti-tumor necrosis factor alpha agent in patients with rheumatoid arthritis: results from a large UK national cohort study. *Arthritis Rheum*. 2007;56:13-20.

[125] Wong PKK, Bagga H, Barrett C, et al. A practical approach to vaccination of patients with autoimmune inflammatory rheumatic diseases in Australia. *Intern Med J*. 2017;47:491-500.

In: Rheumatoid Arthritis
Editor: Amanda Melle
ISBN: 978-1-53613-668-5


*Chapter 2*

# DEPRESSION IN RHEUMATOID ARTHRITIS: SPECIAL CONSIDERATIONS FOR ETHNIC MINORITIES

***Mellissa Withers[1,*], PhD, Patricia Katz[2], MD and George Karpouzas[3], MD***
[1]Keck School of Medicine, University of Southern California, Los Angeles, California, US
[2]Department of Medicine and Institute for Health Policy Studies, University of California San Francisco, San Francisco, California, US
[3]David Geffen School of Medicine, University of California, Los Angeles, California, US

## ABSTRACT

It is increasingly recognized that patients with rheumatoid arthritis (RA) suffer from high rates of depression, which often remains undiagnosed and untreated. In fact, depression was highlighted as the most common comorbidity in a large study on RA patients from 17

---

* Corresponding Author Email: mwithers@usc.edu.

countries. Ethnic minority RA patients are even more likely to experience depression and less likely to seek mental health care than other individuals with RA. Due to its high prevalence and profound impact on functional disability and quality of life, prompt recognition and management of depression is urgently needed in patients with RA, in order to ensure the highest possible physical and mental health and well-being. Rheumatologists will inevitably face the challenge of addressing depression among their patients. In this chapter, we will discuss the prevalence and implications of co-morbid depression in RA patients and sub-groups, focusing on ethnic minorities. We will explore the barriers to identification of depression and the reasons for low utilization of mental health care resources among specific ethnic groups, taking into account patient perceptions of depression and its association with RA. While it is clear that new multidisciplinary clinical protocols should be developed to include depression screening and treatment as part of the rheumatology visit, specific intervention strategies and delivery thereof may differ for diverse ethnic minority groups. We will examine potential intervention approaches, the evidence regarding their effectiveness and cultural acceptability as well as potential for uptake among ethnically diverse patient groups. We will further make recommendations on gaps in education for RA patients with regard to depression. A comprehensive approach to the management of both physical and mental health needs of RA patients can aid in improving patient overall quality of life. Numerous potential strategies could be successfully implemented within the rheumatology clinic setting to better identify co-morbid depression among RA patients generally, and among ethnic minority patients more specifically. Such interventions could help mitigate disability, improve quality of life, patient function and overall satisfaction.

**Keywords:** depression, mental health, race, ethnicity, differences

## Introduction

Depression is defined as a mood disorder with symptoms that include prolonged sadness, loss of interest in daily activities, hopelessness, fatigue, insomnia, and loss of appetite, among others, which last more than two weeks and significantly affect the individual's capacity to function [1]. It is not surprising that many patients who are diagnosed with a serious, long-term condition like RA also suffer from depression. However, depression among persons with RA often remains undiagnosed and untreated.

Depression can have wide-ranging negative consequences in terms of health and daily functioning of RA patients. Ethnic minority patients with RA are even more likely to experience depression and less likely to seek mental health care than other individuals with RA [2]. Due to its high prevalence and profound impact on functional disability and quality of life, prompt recognition and management of depression is urgently needed in patients with RA in order to ensure the highest possible physical and mental health and well-being.

### Chapter Objectives

In this chapter, we review the prevalence of co-morbid depression among RA patients and the range of consequences of depression, focusing on ethnic minority groups. We also analyze the barriers to the identification of depression among RA patients. Finally, we review the evidence on what strategies might be most successful in identifying co-morbid depression within the rheumatology clinic setting in order to effectively manage depression within that setting or through referrals to mental health specialists.

## Prevalence of Depression

The onset of depression often occurs at the time of RA diagnosis [2, 3]. In 2015, 6.7% of adults in the United States (US) reported experiencing depression in the past year [4]. However, among RA patients, studies from around the world have estimated the prevalence of depression among RA patients to be between 9.5% and 41.5%, depending on how depression is defined and measured [5-14]. Studies in the US have estimated a prevalence of between 15-40% among RA patients [2, 3, 15-17].

### Prevalence of Depression among Ethnic Minority Patients

The literature documents higher rates of depression among Hispanic RA patients [2, 16-25]. For example, Karpouzas et al. (2012) reported that 32% of 251 vulnerable US Hispanics with RA from a single center, including 24% of those with low disease activity, had moderate depression levels [23]. Katz et al. (2016) reported a prevalence of 33.8% among Spanish-speaking Hispanic patients in San Francisco [25]. Escalante et al. (2000) documented a depression prevalence of 38-42% among Hispanic RA patients [18]. African American RA patients also experience more depression and report more severe arthritis-related symptoms, such as pain and activity limitations, compared to whites [15, 26]. Morris et al.'s (2011) study of 1,115 RA patients found that intermittent and chronic patterns of depression were far more prevalent among nonwhite participants ($p < .001$) [15]. Less is known about the prevalence of depression among Asian RA patients.

## CONSEQUENCES OF CO-MORBID DEPRESSION IN RA

Depression carries numerous negative implications for RA patients, as well as the overall health system. Depressed RA patients report more severe pain and functional disability [2, 9, 22, 27-44]. Studies have documented reduced pain thresholds among RA patients who are depressed. In turn, depressed RA patients have higher rates of utilization of health services, which results in increased health care costs as compared to non-depressed RA patients [27, 28, 44]. Depression has a significant negative effect on patient global assessment of RA activity jeopardizing attainment or contributing to loss of disease remission. Moreover, depression can contribute to increased disease severity because of noncompliance with treatment [9, 46, 48]. It is further associated with longer hospital stays [9] and ineffective pain management [9, 49]. Moreover, depression has been associated with fatigue, insomnia sleep disturbance [9, 49, 50], myocardial infarction [50], risk of suicide [51, 52], and even death [15, 31, 53-55].

## Synergistic Relationship between RA and Depression

The etiology of depression among RA patients is complex and involves interactions between clinical, demographic, and psychological factors. The relationship between depression and RA is bidirectional and synergistic; the impact of RA on patients' pain and overall functioning can contribute to depression, while depression can also be exacerbated by RA [56, 57]. Depression may lead to increased production of pro-inflammatory cytokines, contributing to an inter-relationship between depression and higher disease activity [55]. There is a clear association between levels of social restriction or isolation, depression, and RA [9, 58, 43, 59, 60]. In a review of 31 studies comprising 16,922 patients with a chronic disease, including diabetes, coronary artery disease, congestive heart failure, asthma, COPD, osteoarthritis, and RA, Katon et al. (2007) showed that when depression or anxiety overlapped with the chronic disease, patients reported a significantly higher number of medical symptoms compared to those with the chronic condition alone, even after controlling for severity of disease. Furthermore, the six studies reviewed relating specifically to RA, showed that severe pain was significantly correlated with depression and anxiety even after controlling for inflammatory markers and demographics [3]. Importantly, depression partially but significantly mediated the effect of pain on functional disability in RA. Covic et al. (2006) reported that depressed RA patients found their RA medication less effective and less important than non-depressed patients. This reduction in perceived treatment effectiveness may lead to treatment non-adherence. In turn, the lack of perceived or actual treatment effectiveness can lead to increases in negative mood [6].

## Functional Disability

Functional problems can be a risk factor for depression; conversely, depression can be a risk factor for functional problems. Considering first the impact of function on depression, Morris et al. (2011) found in a study of 1,115 RA patients over 18 years that greater limitations in basic physical function at baseline were significantly associated with both intermittent and chronic patterns of depression [15]. Margaretten et al. (2009) also found that patients with more reported disability were at greater risk for depression [17]. Katz and Yelin's (2001) study of 654 female RA patients found that loss of recreational and social activities was associated with the subsequent onset of new depressive symptoms. Loss of activities such as hobbies and social interactions were found to be better predictors of depressive symptoms over time than increases in functional limitations, such as grip and bending or stooping [27]. Neugebauer et al. (2003) found that low satisfaction with abilities as a result of RA was the most important predictor of depressive symptoms; the authors wrote that the results underscored "the role of personal meaning attached to changes in functional status in predicting the long-term psychological well-being of individuals with chronic illnesses such as RA" [61].

Depression has also been identified as a predictor of functional disability over time. Increased disability or the loss of function, particularly in valued life activities such as work, social interactions, and family relationships, can translate to diminished overall quality of life for RA patients [9, 29, 38, 59, 60, 62-65]. Michaud and Wolfe (2007) found that patients with both RA and depression are more likely to become work-disabled than patients with RA alone; in fact, depression was *the* most important comorbid condition affecting work-disability in patients with RA [66]. Benka et al. (2016) examined 240 RA patients and found a clear association between levels of social restriction and symptoms of RA; patients with higher restriction levels reported more pain, fatigue, worse functional disability, anxiety, depression, and lower mastery over their disease [43]. Karpouzas et al. (2017) recently reported that presence of depression at baseline was a moderator of significant change in functional disability over time; absence of depression (PHQ9<10) was associated with a significant and clinically meaningful change in disability ($p<0.001$) whereas presence of depression was not ($p=0.12$). Additionally, isolated improvement in PHQ-9 greater than the minimal clinically important difference (MCID) was sufficient and able to independently yield clinically relevant improvement in disability [62]. In the Canadian Community Health Survey, individuals with RA who reported limitations in daily activities were more likely to become depressed [71]. In the study by Covic et al. (2006), depressed RA patients experienced significantly higher levels of perceived changes in functioning due to RA compared to non-depressed patients, particularly relating to levels of physical and recreational changes. Fifty percent of depressed patients reported experiencing significant physical changes, such as joint deformation and weight fluctuations, and 61% experienced significant changes in recreational activities [6].

## Pain

Pain is a well-documented risk factor for depression. For example, Morris found that higher ratings of pain were significantly associated with subsequent depression [15]. Similarly, individuals with RA in the Canadian Community Health Survey who had chronic pain were more likely to become depressed [67]. Wolfe and Michaud (2009) found that a combined measurement of fatigue and widespread pain was the most important predictor of depression among RA patients [16]. Conversely, depression can increase sensitivity to pain and decrease pain thresholds.

## Psychological Factors

Depression and its associated impairments can contribute to feelings of helplessness, pessimistic outlook, or perceived lack of control over pain or RA [6]. For example, studies have demonstrated an association between depression and disease acceptance and/or perception of the severity of the disease among patients with RA. Furthermore, the level of functioning and overall quality of life of RA patients may be associated with psychological characteristics and is not predicted by disease burden alone. For example, Ormseth and colleagues study (2015) used cross-sectional baseline data from RA patients who participated in a clinical trial comparing behavioral treatments for RA: the results showed that adjustment to RA was highly individualized [65], confirming other studies that have shown that psychological variables predict role functioning in RA independently of pain and disease activity [12, 16, 34, 35]. Pinto-Gouveia et al. (2013) found that subjects who had better disease acceptance reported less pain, fewer physical limitations, and lower overall depression levels. Importantly, they noted that patients with higher level of disease acceptance were less likely to develop depression [68]. Rezai et al. (2014) found in their study of 100 RA patients in Iran that higher depression symptoms were associated with increased perceived pain, more negative illness perceptions, greater functional impairment, graver perceived consequences and less control over the disease [42]. The results suggested that the relationship between depression symptoms and pain were partially mediated by illness perception. The term "catastrophizing" is defined by a specific set of cognitive and emotional responses to pain, such as the degree to which a patient feels helpless when in pain, the tendency to ruminate about pain, and the propensity of magnify the threat value of pain [69-72]. In their review of 10 published articles relating to pain catastrophizing and depression among patients with chronic conditions, Edwards et al. (2011) found that in patients with RA, catastrophizing and depression were linked to increased pain, higher reported physical self-limitation, reduced likelihood of returning to work, less exercise, fewer health-promoting behaviors, lower thresholds and tolerance to pain, and more difficulties suppressing thoughts of pain [72]. Treharne et al. (2005) examined the relationships of psychosocial factors with well-being in RA patients. Fifty-five patients with early RA (< six months), 52 with intermediate duration RA (one-seven years) and 47 with established

RA (> seven years) were surveyed on psychosocial factors and psychological and physical well-being. Illness perceptions related to worse depression and life satisfaction, especially among newly diagnosed patients. Optimism related to lower pain in early and intermediate RA and social support was associated with less reported fatigue in patients with established RA [73].

### Other Factors

Other health problems, particularly more serious comorbidities, increase the likelihood of depression [15, 67]. A number of sociodemographic factors also increase the risk of depression. In addition to racial/ethnic status, other demographic characteristics that are associated with depression among RA patients include female sex [14, 18, 74-77], younger age [9, 58, 78-80], lower socioeconomic status [6, 15, 27, 28, 77-81] and single marital status [77, 79].

## Diagnosing Depression in the Rheumatology Clinic

Diagnosis of depression represents an important way that rheumatologists can work to improve RA patients' quality of life. In fact, clinically meaningful improvement in depression has been shown to independently predict equally relevant improvement in disability [62]. Many studies have highlighted the challenge of identification and management of depression within the rheumatology clinic, recognizing that identification of depression among RA patients may be hindered by both patient-level and systems-level barriers [56, 82].

At a patient-level, the range and continuum of depressive symptoms may not be well-understood. Even when RA patients recognize the symptoms of depression, they may be reluctant to mention depression to rheumatologists because of time constraints, lack of provider continuity, perceived stigma around the symptoms, or because they feel that depressive symptoms are only appropriate to mention with mental health providers [2]. Depressive symptoms may also appear clinically very similar to symptoms of RA, and patients may misattribute their symptoms to RA, therefore not recognizing the problem [56, 83].

Most rheumatologists do not routinely screen their RA patients for depression due to time constraints, inadequate referral services, lack of training and confidence in dealing with mental health issues, or the belief that mental health care professionals should handle mental health issues among RA patients [56, 83, 84]. Sleath et al. (2008) reported that less than one in five severely depressed RA patients (PHQ-9>15) had the opportunity to discuss their depression during rheumatology clinic visits. Even when depression was addressed, the discussion was initiated by the patient and was fairly limited; not once during the 200 observed office visits did a rheumatologist bring up the topic of depression to the patient. They found that patients were significantly more likely to disclose psychological distress if physicians asked about it, if there was greater physician-patient familiarity, and if there was greater severity of psychological distress. Disclosure was significantly related to providers' recognition of the mental health problem [82].

Rheumatology is not unique in the lack of attention to depression. Studies have shown that depression screening is generally low within the primary care setting. Sleath and Rubin (2002) found that depression was discussed during only 25% of 383 primary care visits. Patients who rated their emotional health poorly were significantly more likely to discuss depression. Patients initiated the discussion regarding depression 55% of the time. Female patients and patients who were more educated were significantly more likely to raise the topic of depression before their physicians did [84].

## Treatment of Depression among RA Patients

Depression is a treatable disorder and the efficacy of pharmacological, psychological, and behavioral treatments for depression are well-documented.

### Pharmacological Treatments

Antidepressant medication has shown great success in treating some depressed patients. Clarke and Currie's (2009) systematic literature review of 159 published articles from 1995 to 2007 found that, of the small number of studies dealing with antidepressants as treatment, medication was an effective treatment option for depressed RA patients [9]. Fiest et al. (2017) examined eight controlled trials conducted in persons with RA and depression or anxiety; they concluded that the level of evidence was low to moderate due to risk of bias and small numbers. Among six pharmacological interventions for depression, the three with active comparators did improve depressive symptoms [85].

### Psychological Treatments

Emotional regulation process involves focusing on the present, which is perceived to promote change in the way that symptoms are experienced, emphasizing the relationship between body, thoughts and emotions [86-92]. Pain acceptance has been related to improvements in how patients react and adapt to chronic pain [92, 93]. It is concerned with engagement in life activities while in pain, and the recognition that attempts to control or avoid pain are ineffective strategies [89, 93, 94]. Acceptance has been associated with better emotional, physical, social and work-related functioning, as well as less use of health-care resources [87-90]. Individuals who recognize their pain and physical limitations, but act as if these did not necessarily imply disability, live more fulfilling lives [87-94]. Pinto-Gouveia et al.'s (2013) study suggested that an attitude of willingness to face unwanted internal experiences at the early stages of the RA influenced the level of pain and physical limitation reported by patients during the progression of the disease. Patients with low levels of acceptance and low social support had more depression, which was perceived to be due to patients' self-evaluation as disabled, limited or dependent. The authors reported "results also showed that participants with higher scores of willingness to perform daily activities and who recognized the ineffectiveness of attempts to control or avoid unwanted internal experiences reported lower depressive symptoms at the baseline assessment. Moreover, the negative association of acceptance and the rate of depression growth showed that participants with higher levels of acceptance between the baseline and the following two years presented a lower rate of depression growth over time. One possible mechanism of the association between depression and acceptance might be the fact that acceptance promotes the contact with the present moment, allowing the individual to take better advantage of its positive processes such as the interactions with family members" [68]. It should be noted, however, that the one psychological treatment included in Fiest's (2017) review of controlled trial did not improve depressive symptoms [85].

## Behavioral Treatments

Behavioral interventions have shown some promise in helping RA patients to cope with their disease-related impairments and negative emotional states that may interfere with quality of life. Garfenski et al. (2013) reported on an internet-based cognitive behavioral self-help intervention on depression, anxiety, and coping self-efficacy in people with RA. The program, which included components of relaxation, changing maladaptive cognitions, and attainment of personal life goals, incorporated minimal outside coaching. After only a two-month follow-up period, the intervention significantly improved depression and anxiety and strengthened coping self-efficacy in RA patients. Enhancing coping self-efficacy may be valuable in helping RA patients to adjust to and cope with lifelong RA-related impairments [93-95].

Mindfulness meditation has been proven effective in several studies to help RA patients manage or overcome depression [6, 96, 97]. Pradhan et al. (2007) found mindfulness meditation to be effective in alleviating psychological distress in RA patients [96]. Zautra et al. (2008) found that both cognitive behavioral therapy and affective interventions (such as mindfulness meditation and emotional regulation therapy) reduced depression among RA patients [97].

In general population studies, physical activity and exercise interventions show positive effects on depression. The American Psychiatric Associated even recommends physical activity as beneficial for depression, particularly among individuals with co-occurring medical problems. Physical activity and exercise also hold promise in reducing depression among RA patients [98-101]. A Cochrane review found physical activity interventions were as effective as psychological or pharmacological therapy in treating depression [100]. Neuberger et al. (2007) found that exercise had a positive influence on depression in a randomized trial of 220 RA patients. Patients were randomized to class exercises, home exercises using videotapes, and the control group. After 12 weeks of exercise, the class exercise group had a statistically significant difference in overall symptoms (including depression) as compared to the control group [98]. Herring et al. (2012) conducted a systematic review of 90 randomized, controlled studies evaluating the impact of exercise on participants with chronic diseases. The results demonstrated that physical exercise was related to a significant reduction in depressive symptoms among patients with chronic disease and the largest reduction of depressive symptoms came from patients with moderately elevated depressive symptoms at baseline [99]. Kelley's (2016) review of 29 published studies that included 2,449 participants (1460 exercise and 979 control) with RA and other rheumatic diseases found that 51.7% of the studies evaluating the effects of exercise on depressive symptoms had results that were statistically significant ($p<0.05$) [101]. Middleton et al. (2013) reported that there is promising evidence that yoga therapy may help both osteoarthritis and rheumatoid arthritis [102].

Emotional and peer support can also have a significant positive impact on depression [21, 32]. Neugebauer and Katz (2004) found that emotional support had a significant short-term impact on depression, although it may not be able to overcome the impact of functional disability on future depression [36]. The use of peers or community health workers may be effective in increasing knowledge help-seeking behaviors and health outcomes, particularly among racial/ethnic minorities [103-105]. Hansen and Cabassa et al. (2010) and others [106-108] have reported external recognition, such as by family and friends, are important in the recognition of the need for depression treatment, as well as initiation of treatment. They highlighted how help-seeking often begins within family unit and expands out when the situation deteriorates or care within this intimate network is exhausted or not provided. Close family and friends may be able to call the patient's attention to changes in behavior or emotions and promote help-seeking behavior. The lack of support from family or friends may necessitate that patients expand help-seeking to outsiders, which delays care. Encouraging patients with spiritual beliefs to seek support from their churches or religious networks may also be helpful.

## Treatment Preferences among Racial/Ethnic Minority RA Patients

Several studies have examined racial/ethnic differences in treatment preferences and have found that racial/ethnic minorities often prefer psychological counseling over antidepressant medication [3, 18, 106-113]. Karasz and Watkins (2006) found that Hispanic patients felt that both antidepressants and counseling would be helpful treatments, but that counseling would be more helpful [114]. Cooper et al. (2003) found

Hispanic and white patients were generally accepting of both counseling and antidepressants, but that Hispanic patients were less accepting of antidepressants and more accepting of counseling. African Americans were the least likely to find antidepressant medication acceptable [111]. In a study by Withers et al. exploring depression awareness, barriers to disclosure and treatment options in Hispanics with RA, antidepressants were not acceptable; they were viewed as unnecessary, harmful, highly addictive, life-long treatments, fraught with side effects [2]. The majority stated they would be willing, or at least not opposed, to seeing a therapist if necessary. Depression was viewed as a condition not successfully treated by medication. Since depression was associated with personal weakness and character flaws, the theme of self-reliance, self-treatment, and personal strength emerged repeatedly. Positive thinking was perceived as the most important treatment for depression. Givens et al.'s (2007) study of 78,753 patients with depression, including 3596 African Americans, 2794 Asians/Pacific Islanders and 3203 Hispanics, found that racial/ethnic minority patients were more likely to prefer counseling to medications as compared to whites (African Americans (OR)=2.6, 95% 95% CI=2.4-2.8), Asians/Pacific Islanders (OR=2.5, 95% CI=2.2-2.7) and Hispanics (OR=1.8, 95% CI=1.7-2.0). The racial/ethnic minority patients were less likely to believe that medications were effective and that depression was biologically based, but were more likely to believe that antidepressants were addictive. They were also more likely to believe that counseling and prayer were effective [109]. Religious coping, such as faith in God and prayer, as help for depression has been documented as potentially effective among racial/ethnic minorities [18]. Cabassa et al. (2007) found that psychotherapy is also congruent with the Hispanic cultural value of "*desahogarse*" (unburdening), providing a safe context where participants could unburden their problems and receive advice and support from a trusted individual [108].

## Barriers to Identification and Treatment of Depression among Racial/Ethnic Minority RA Patients

While barriers to identification and treatment for depression exist for RA patients in general, some are particularly relevant for racial/ethnic minorities.

### Systems-Level Barriers

Racial/ethnic minorities may encounter a multitude of systems-level barriers to disclosure of depression, including lack of language-matched providers or the lack of access to psychotherapy services [3, 23-25, 77, 106, 107]. Withers et al. (2016) found systems-related barriers, such as lack of English fluency or language-matched providers, were major barriers to depression disclosure among Hispanic patients. While translators were available and many providers spoke rudimentary Spanish, Hispanic RA patients did not feel these overcame communication difficulties. Participants also associated rheumatology appointments with physical illness and did not initiate discussion of mental health issues, citing provider responsibility to raise the topic of depression. Little education was given to patients regarding depression, and poor awareness regarding the range of symptoms of depression also inhibited patient recognition of depression [2].

### Patient-Provider Relationships and Communication

Studies among racial/ethnic minority patients with RA have demonstrated that the patient-provider relationship is extremely important in determining whether patients will seek mental health care [2, 13, 18, 21, 115]. Berrios-Rivera et al. (2006) examined the role of trust in patient–

physician relationships among 70 RA and 32 lupus patients, of which 25% were white, 43% were Latino, and 31% were African-American. About three-quarters of the sample was female. On average, patients rated their perceptions of medical interaction and trust in their physician as moderately positive. Scores on informative nature, sensitivity to concerns, reassurance and support, patient-centeredness, and participatory decision-making were all highly positively correlated with trust in the physician. Lower trust in physicians was observed in Latino and African-American patients, as compared with white patients. Physicians who focused on patients' concerns had more effective patient communication. Trust in the U.S. health care system was an independent predictor of trust in physicians. The authors hypothesized that differences in communication styles, subconscious biases, stereotypes, and misconceptions may have impeded effective communication, empathy, and trust between patients and physicians [115]. Withers et al. (2016) reported that only one-quarter of Hispanic RA patients in their sample who were currently depressed had disclosed depression to their providers. Most participants did not see the same rheumatologist regularly and did not feel they had established relationship of trust that would encourage communication about depression. Additionally, short time for clinic interaction with providers inhibited the ability to form this relationship, and inhibited disclosure of depression. Patients generally believed that such discussions should be initiated by providers because they felt that depressed people were not likely to discuss their condition with others, including health care providers and, even family members [2]. Hansen and Cabassa (2012) found in their study of help-seeking experiences of low-income Latinos with diabetes and depression that having a trusting relationship with their provider enhanced motivation to take antidepressant medications and/or attend therapy sessions. The authors explained that "participants' evaluations of how their treatment contributed to alleviation of symptoms and improvement in functioning were linked to adherence behaviors. These findings suggest that individuals' subjective experiences of treatment, particularly perceived treatment benefits, evolved through the course of treatment and played a role in shaping adherence" [108].

"*Respeto*" is an important value among Hispanics that relates to the hierarchical structures that may exist in Hispanic communities, which may contribute to deferential behaviors toward others based on age, gender, social or economic status, authority, or other characteristics. This value often is associated with respect and obedience towards elders or people in positions of authority. Studies have documented that Hispanics may not feel it is appropriate to question or defy physicians' authority, which may lead to lack of patient-provider communications, misunderstandings, or non-compliance [2, 108, 106, 107]. Cabassa et al. (2007) found that depressive symptoms were related to patients' attitudes toward their doctors' interpersonal skills. The author suggested that "depressive symptoms, through their impact on patients' attitudes, may interfere with the development of a trusting doctor-patient relationship, possibly hindering the identification and treatment of depression. In addition, patients' distrust of physicians and their skepticism toward the effectiveness of antidepressants may act as barriers for seeking professional care and adhering to treatment" [108].

## Stigma

Another important barrier to mental health help-seeking among racial/ethnic minorities is the stigma associated with mental illness [106, 108, 116]. In Vega et al.'s study (2010), 200 low-income, Spanish-speaking, Latino patients in primary care clinics were screened for depression and completed a stigma checklist. Patients reporting higher levels of perceived stigma were less likely to disclose their depression diagnosis to their family and friends, less likely to be taking depression medication (OR=.78; 95% CI, .62-.99), less likely to be able to manage their depression (OR=.79; 95% CI, .65-.96) and more likely to have missed scheduled appointment visits (OR=1.44; 95% CI, 1.03-2.02) [116]. Patients' reluctance to discuss their depressive symptoms with others, which may be related to uncertainty about the cause of their symptoms, negative attitudes towards mental illness, or not wanting to worry family about their needs, can delay treatment initiation [106].

The belief that illness, particularly mental illness, is related to personal weakness also contributes to stigma. Studies have found that depression is often associated with weakness, bad habits, personal failures, or character flaws, such as drinking or spending money frivolously [6, 106, 117]. Some racial/ethnic minority patients believe that depressed people had the power to prevent, or at least recover from, depression on their own. Such attitudes of self-reliance, control, and self-management of depression have been found to influence health seeking behavior in other studies among Hispanics [2, 13, 18, 106-108, 118, 119]. Withers et al. (2016) reported that the theme of self-reliance, self-treatment and personal strength came up repeatedly in their interviews with Hispanic RA patients. Positive thinking was believed to be the *most* important treatment for depression, and most felt that people who demonstrated a positive attitude and strength of character could triumph over depression. Most felt that an individual could overcome depression simply with one's own will to get better [2].

## Fear of Medications

A barrier to antidepressant use among racial/ethnic minorities is the fear of side effects, especially addiction [2, 18, 106-108]. Withers et al. (2016) found that Hispanics viewed anti-depressants as unnecessary, harmful, highly addictive, having negative side effects, and need to be used life-long. Some viewed depression a condition that could not be treated successfully with medication. Some felt that depression was an expected result of having a chronic disease, and was a normal part of the RA trajectory versus a separate illness that could be treated within a health care setting [2]. Hansen and Cabassa (2012) also found that antidepressants were viewed as addictive and harmful, and patients feared being labeled as crazy if they took them [106]. Other studies have also found that stigma may play an important role in the low utilization of mental health services among racial/ethnic minorities, as well as negatively impact initiation and adherence to antidepressant treatment [116, 120, 121].

## Social Stressors

The literature also sheds light on the association between depression and general social stressors that may be particularly relevant for racial/ethnic minorities. It may be useful to examine the contextual factors of patients' lives that influence quality of life and may enhance risk of depression. Social stressors such as family dynamics, working conditions, and financial challenges may relate to RA and depression outcomes. Conversely, patients may be better able to manage disease if these stressors are addressed. For example, immigrants may face hardships relating to social isolation, lack of family and social support, discrimination, few employment opportunities, and long work hours or low wages that may increase risk of depression [77]. Social stressors such as economic strains, employment issues, and caregiving responsibilities play an important role in patients' explanatory models of the causes of depression [68-70]. Thus, failure to acknowledge these social stressors may alienate patients, discourage them from engaging in treatments, or lead to low adherence to care [107].

## Acculturation

The level of acculturation of immigrant patients may also play an important role in help-seeking behaviors, risk of depression, and overall health outcomes [2, 108, 117, 122, 123]. Hispanics and Asians are often lumped into single categories but important differences may exist within each group by place of birth, language abilities, or level of acculturation. For example, Lackey et al. (2013) and Escalante et al. (2000) highlighted differences in care between native-born and foreign-born Latinos [18, 124]. Katz et al. (2016) found that Hispanic RA patients who were fluent in English did not have significantly different disease status from white patient, and both groups had better outcomes than Hispanic patients who were not fluent in English. In other words, the effects of ethnicity appeared to be outweighed by the effects of sociodemographic factors or other cultural factors. The prevalence of depression in the Spanish-speaking Hispanic group was also twice that of both the white and English-speaking Hispanic groups [25].

## Racial/Ethnic Disparities in Care, Treatment, and Outcomes That May Influence Depression

The literature has documented numerous disparities in healthcare access, treatment, and outcomes among racial/ethnic minority RA patients as compared to white RA patients that may influence the risk of depression or the consequences of comorbid depression. Racial/ethnic minorities may be particularly vulnerable to the synergistic relationship between RA and depression because of a greater likelihood of having other risk factors for depression, such as low socioeconomic status or social stressors [18, 25, 77]. For example, low socioeconomic status is significantly related to poorer disease outcomes in African Americans, particularly patient-reported outcomes such as health status, pain and fatigue [125]. Low social position in both childhood and adulthood has been linked with poor RA outcomes, including laboratory and radiographic RA disease severity measures and patient-reported outcomes, in African-Americans [126]. Spanish-speaking Hispanic RA patients have been found to have worse function, higher levels of pain, and to be more likely to have moderate to severe fatigue than English-proficient groups of whites and Hispanics [25]. In the study, the authors reasoned that sociodemographic differences played a significant role in explaining disparities in these outcomes, as large differences existed in terms of sociodemographic characteristics of the Spanish-speaking Hispanic group as compared to the English-proficient groups. Monolingual Spanish speakers had lower education and income levels, low health literacy, were more likely have no health insurance or Medicaid, and were less likely to have been born in the US. Low education and low income accounted for some of the differences in health outcomes, including daily functioning, between the Spanish- and English-speaking groups [25]. Cabassa et al.'s (2007) study showed that Hispanic patients attributed depression to life circumstances and social pressures, such as interpersonal difficulties, financial strains, and stress rather than to internal mechanisms related to biological, genetic or chemical factors. Patients also lacked emotional support system to help them cope with these life circumstances and difficulties [108]. These "situational" or contextual models of depression among racial/ethnic minorities have been reported by others [2, 114, 127].

Several studies have found that racial/ethnic minority RA patients report greater disability, more pain and fatigue, less effective drug therapy, lower adherence to therapy, and worse disease activity and overall health status [128-131]. For example, in a cross-sectional study of 4,730 RA patients, of which 91% were white and 76% were female, whites were found to be significantly older and better educated than African Americans and Hispanics, and had their RA longer (16 vs 13 and 15 yrs), yet had the least amount of disability and the best health status, as compared with the other racial/ethnic groups. African-Americans reported the most pain but Hispanics also scored higher in pain scores than whites. Factors related to pain among African-Americans and Hispanics included education, disease duration, and other chronic comorbidities [20].

Unique factors may also influence RA outcomes in racial/ethnic minority groups. McIlvane et al. [129, 130] examined differences in stress and outcomes among 77 African American women and 98 white women with RA. African American women reported more functional impairment, life stressors, financial stress, and discrimination, but lower perceived arthritis stress. There were no differences between the groups in depression, although the factors associated with depression differed. Chronic life stressors played a greater role in depression for African American women, including perceptions of greater stress due to arthritis, financial stress, and everyday discrimination. In contrast, functional impairment was related to higher depressive symptoms for white women.

The literature has also documented differences in initiation of drug therapy for RA [131, 132] and adherence to RA medication [133, 134] between racial/ethnic minorities and whites. For example, in a study among ethnic minority RA patients in public and private clinics in Texas, racial/ethnic minority patients were less than half as likely to receive a drug for RA and had a significantly increased length of time to drug initiation versus whites (median of 7 years versus median of 1 year) [132]. These racial and ethnic disparities in initiation of drug therapy suggested that these populations did not receive appropriate and timely treatment for RA, which could have both short-term and long-term health impacts. In a cross-sectional survey of 102 patients, including 70 with RA, of which 43% were Hispanic, 32% were African-American, and 25% were white, one quarter of racial/ethnic minority patients had adherence problems to their medication, as compared to only 11% of whites. The five most commonly cited reasons were feeling like the drug was toxic/harmful, sleeping through the dose time, feeling sick or ill, feeling depressed or overwhelmed, or having problems taking pills at specified times [133].

## Recommendations

Depression negatively impacts the health and well-being of RA patients. Therefore, new protocols for the identification and management of depression within the rheumatology clinic setting could help management of RA, as well as improve patients' overall quality of life. We suggest ten key strategies that can be implemented within the clinical setting to improve identification and management of depression in RA patients.

1) Early diagnosis and treatment of depression could help to promote optimal health and resilience. Patients may be at highest risk of depression at the time of RA diagnosis [21, 33, 56]. Rheumatologists and health care providers should be cognizant of this high-risk time period so that they can be watchful of any depressive symptoms among newly-diagnosed RA patients. Furthermore, patients that have highest risk of depression, such as

females, younger patients, and those from racial/ethnic minority groups, should be carefully monitored for depressive symptoms.

2) Providing patients and their families with education about depression and how to identify the symptoms as early as possible after diagnosis is critical in order to improve the likelihood of self-identification of early depressive symptoms. Increased awareness can help prepare patients and their families for the risk of depression and how to recognize it. This may also help address misconceptions and knowledge gaps regarding depression, as well as reduce stigma associated with depression. Patients should be made aware of the association between RA and depression, and that many of the symptoms of depression may mimic RA. It is also important that they understand the range of potential symptoms, and the varying degrees of severity that patients who are depressed may experience. Raising public awareness about the increased risk of depression among patients suffering from RA and other chronic conditions could also help promote more help-seeking behaviors among patients, as well as potentially reduce community-level stigma associated with mental health issues.
3) Stigma associated with depression and other mental health issues is a major barrier to effective management of depression. Increasing awareness regarding symptom continuum and range of experiences that depressed people incur may lead to both earlier recognition and stigma reduction. Rectifying misconceptions about depression's relation to personal character flaws or bad habits might eliminate the blame bestowed upon depressed individuals, motivating more to seek treatment.
4) Routine screening for depression should be implemented in rheumatology clinics. Empirically validated diagnostic procedures exist for identifying and managing depression. Such tools can be self-administered by patients within a relatively short timeframe. For example, the Patient Health Questionnaire (PHQ9) provides cutoff scores that have high specificity and sensitivity for detecting depression. However, verbal screening by health care providers

may yield higher disclosure rates [2, 26, 27, 28, 29]. Yet, screening is not routinely implemented in rheumatology practice, highlighting an important service delivery gap in clinical care [56]. Screening mechanisms should be implemented beginning at the time of RA diagnosis and screening should continue on a regular basis to assess depression over the course of a patient's care, even after the symptoms of RA are under control. The Canadian Dermatology-Rheumatology Comorbidity Initiative recommended more awareness of among healthcare providers with regard to the heightened risk of depression among RA patients, as well as the implementation of screening. They also advised that providers should be aware of the synergistic relationship between RA and depression, specifically that symptoms of depression may affect disease activity measures and that disease symptoms may also affect depression scores [57].

5) RA patients should also be encouraged to discuss mental health issues with their rheumatologists, and providers should be proactive in initiating such discussions. Patients may be unwilling to initiate discussions about mental health issues; therefore, providers should take a more active role in initiating such discussions. Health care providers should assess patients' negative attitudes toward depression and treatment options in order to mitigate potential barriers to care and engage patients in effective treatment. Providers should be aware of the potential influence of cultural beliefs on attitudes and mental health seeking-behaviors in patients. In particular, providers can play an important role in addressing any doubts, concerns, or misconceptions regarding the effectiveness and potential side effects of antidepressants.
6) Rheumatologists should incorporate depression identification and management plan into patient care plans. For example, if screening scores suggest mild depression, psychological intervention may not be necessary but follow-up is needed to determine if the depression worsens over time. However, if the scores demonstrate that the patient is likely experiencing a more serious depressive

disorder, consultation with a mental health professional is necessary. Clinical psychologists or psychiatrists who have training in understanding the relationship between psychological factors and chronic disease are the most qualified to address mental health problems among patients and to coordinate care plans with rheumatologists [57]. A timely referral system should be established for patients who need to consult with a mental health professional who could give a definitive diagnosis and establish a management approach. Regular communication between the rheumatologist and mental health professional is required in order to effectively manage both issues.

7) Consideration of a holistic approach to patient overall well-being and functioning is important. This necessitates examining more than just the management of pain; for patients, the perception of disability may involve much more than simply the absence of pain [19]. While disease control may reduce symptoms of depression among RA patients, patients' own perceptions of RA, such as their level of impairment and the impact it has on daily functioning, are critical in terms of both their physical and mental health outcomes. For example, regardless of actual disease activity, studies have shown that patients who perceive lower levels of control over their conditions may feel more helplessness, which can contribute to higher rates of depression [39]. Social stressors and contextual factors in patients' lives that heighten depression risk should also be taken into consideration.
8) Providing patients with information about resources to help them develop coping strategies could reduce the risk depression. This type of information should be provided soon after diagnosis of RA, along with strong encouragement to engage these resources, in order to prevent depression or lessen its impact if patients experience depressive symptoms. Resilience and mastery over illness have been found to be critical in terms of helping RA patients overcome depression [40]. Neugebauer et al. (2003) highlighted the role that changes in functional status have in

predicting the long-term psychological well-being of individuals with chronic illnesses and found that the maintenance of valued activities is a critical factor in the psychological adjustment of RA patients [61]. More research is needed on the lived experiences of the patient and the personal meaning of their disease.

9) Physical activity and social participation are also essential to patients' mental health and can improve depressive symptoms. Patients should be encouraged to participate in as many daily activities as possible. Studies have also highlighted the association and synergies between depression and the impact of RA in terms of impairment and daily functioning and have found that fewer restrictions and higher maintenance of social participation can help reduce depression among RA patients [32, 39, 43, 61]. Support groups run by peers or health professionals may have utility in helping patients cope with RA and/or depression [2, 21]. Interventions that incorporate exercise or physical activity for RA patients are also recommended, as these can be effective in improving depression [98-101].
10) Sociocultural factors also have an important influence RA and depression outcomes in racial/ethnic minority patients. In order to successfully manage comorbid depression among RA among racial/ethnic minority patients, who suffer a greater burden of depression, establishing which strategies would be culturally acceptable, relevant, and effective for the identification and management of depression and how to best deliver them is needed. Racial/ethnic minority patients also face unique barriers to care, including socioeconomic challenges to accessing care and language and literacy barriers in communicating with physicians or understanding treatments. For example, language barriers can negatively impact quality of care and increase disparities in health outcomes. Limited English abilities may hinder scheduling appointments, as well as patient-provider interactions during clinic visits. Patients with limited English proficiency can benefit from bilingual providers or interpreters who are readily available to

interact with patients and providers. Cultural factors can also influence communication with physicians, perceptions of disease, and willingness or ability to accept or adhere to treatments [106]. Sensitivity to these cultural issues can facilitate acceptance, adherence, and ultimately success of any depression intervention. Strategies might include incorporation of culturally relevant references, assessment and tailoring of depression education on a patient level, exploration and understanding of cultural and personal beliefs around potential reasons for depression incidence and intensity, and ultimately fostering and building on attitudes of self-resilience and self-reliance [21].

## CONCLUSION

Depression often remains undiagnosed and untreated among RA patients, especially racial/ethnic minorities. Rheumatologists face a major challenge of addressing depression in their clinical interactions with patients. Due to the high prevalence, the wide range of negative consequences, cyclical nature, and the documented synergistic relationship between RA and depression, evaluating and addressing comorbid depression is an essential part of RA care. A comprehensive approach to the management of both physical and mental health needs of RA patients is likely to yield the best health outcomes. Clinical protocols should include routine depression screening as part of the rheumatology visit. Additional educational efforts for patients and their families are needed to address misconceptions and knowledge gaps, as well as reduce stigma associated with depression. More counseling resources are also needed to provide treatment for those suffering from depression, which could help mitigate disability, improve quality of life, patient function and overall satisfaction.

Socioeconomic and racial/ethnic disparities exist in treating depression among RA patients, stemming from variety of complex factors, including systems-related factors, such as clinic practices and patient-provider communication, as well as individual-level factors, such as treatment preferences, health literacy, and cultural beliefs. Despite the high prevalence of depression among racial/ethnic minorities with RA, little is known about their awareness and perceptions of the etiology and manifestations of depressive symptoms and its association with RA. More research is needed on depression among racial/ethnic minorities with RA, including what role of sociocultural factors may play in the identification of depression and culturally-appropriate interventions. Data from large studies should be disaggregated to examine different characteristics of racial/ethnic minority groups in order to better understand their needs. For example, Hispanics who are foreign-born may exhibit very different patterns of behavior and risk factors for depression than Hispanics born in the US. Development of intervention approaches specifically for RA patients from racial/ethnic minorities that are realistic given the constraints within the healthcare setting and the patients' own unique challenges is critical to delivering appropriate care. While the content of CBT interventions has been developed and validated for racial/ethnic minorities, the delivery of such information should also be tailored to fit the needs of racial/ethnic minority patients with a chronic condition like RA [10, 19, 20]. Focusing on culturally meaningful themes such as coping strategies, stress reduction techniques, positive thinking, self-efficacy, self-esteem, and resiliency may facilitate uptake, adherence and successful outcome [10, 19, 20].

## REFERENCES

[1] American Psychiatric Association (APA). (2013) *Diagnostic and Statistical Manual of Mental Disorders*-Fifth Edition. Accessed 19 April 2017 at: http://dsm.psychiatryonline.org/doi/book/10.1176/appi.books.9780890425596.

[2] Withers M, Moran R, Nicassio P, Weisman M, Karpouzas G. Perspectives of vulnerable Hispanics with rheumatoid arthritis on depression: Awareness, Barriers to Disclosure, and Treatment Options. *Arthritis Care Res* 2015;67:484-492.

[3] Katon W, Lin E, Kroenkem K. The association of depression and anxiety with medical symptom burden in patients with chronic medical illness. *General Hospital Psychiatry* 2007;29:147-155.

[4] U.S. National Institute of Mental Health. *2015 National Survey on Drug Use and Health* (*NSDUH*). Accessed 25 May 2017 at: https://www.nimh.nih.gov/health/topics/depression/index.shtml.

[5] Dickens CA, McGowan L, Clark-Carter D, et al. Depression in rheumatoid arthritis: a systematic review of the literature with meta-analysis. *Psychosom Med.* 2002, 64:52-60.

[6] Covic T, Tyson G, Spencer D, Howe G. Depression in rheumatoid arthritis patients: demographic, clinical, and psychological predictors. *Journal of Psychosomatic Research.* 2006;60:469-476.

[7] Nicassio PM, Understanding the role and significance of gender differences in pain and depression in Chinese elders with osteoarthritis. *Pain.* 2007;130:6-7.

[8] Isik A, Koca, SS, Ozturk, A, Mermi, O. Anxiety and depression in patients with rheumatoid arthritis. *Clin Rheumatol.* 2007;26:872-878.

[9] Clarke DM, Currie, KC. Depression, anxiety, and their relationship with chronic diseases: A review of the epidemiology, risk, and treatment evidence. *Med J of Australia* 2009;191:S54-S60.

[10] Lok EYC, Mok CC, Cheng CW, Cheung EFC. Prevalence and determinants of psychiatric disorders in patients with rheumatoid arthritis. *Psychosomatics*. 2010;51:338-U120.

[11] Matcham F, Rayner L, Steer S, Hotopf M. The prevalence of depression in rheumatoid arthritis: a systematic review and meta-analysis. *Rheumatology*. 2013;52:2136-2148.

[12] Dougados M, Perrodeau E, Fayet F, et al. Impact of a nurse led program of patient self-assessment of disease activity on the management of rheumatoid arthritis: Results of a prospective, multicentre, randomized, control trial (COMEDRA). *Annals of the Rheumatic Diseases.* 2013;72:150.

[13] Eusden J, Matcham F, Hotopf M, et al. The relationship between mental health, disease severity, and genetic disorders in early

rheumatoid arthritis. *Psychosomatic Medicine* 2017. Accessed 29 April 2017 at: http://insights.ovid.com/crossref?an=00006842-900000000-98839.

[14] Maiden NL, Hurst NP, Lochhead A, Carson AJ, Sharpe M. Quantifying the burden of emotional ill-health amongst patients referred to a specialist rheumatology service. *Rheumatology.* 2003;42:750-7.

[15] Morris A, Yelin EH, Panopalis P, et al. Long-term patterns of depression and associations with health and function in a panel study of rheumatoid arthritis. *J Health Psychol.* 2011;16:667-77.

[16] Wolfe K, Michaud, K. Predicting depression in rheumatoid arthritis: The signal importance of pain extent and fatigue, and comorbidity. *Arthritis and Rheumatism.* 2009;61:667-673.

[17] Margaretten M, Yelin E, Imboden J, et al. Predictors of depression in a multiethnic cohort of patients with rheumatoid arthritis. *Arthritis Rheumatology* 2009;61:1586-1591.

[18] Escalante A, Rincon I, Mulrow CD. Symptoms of depression and psychological distress among Hispanics with rheumatoid arthritis. *Arthritis Care Res.* 2000;13:156-167.

[19] Del Rincon I, Battafarano DF, Arroyo RA, Murphy FT, Fischbach M, Escalante A. Ethnic variation in the clinical manifestations of rheumatoid arthritis: role of HLA-DRB1 alleles. *Arthritis Rheum.* 2003;49:200-208.

[20] Bruce B, Fries JF, Murtagh KN. Health status disparities in ethnic minority patients with rheumatoid arthritis: a cross-sectional study. *J Rheumatol.* 2007;34:1475–9.

[21] Yazici Y, Kautiainen H, Sokka T. Differences in clinical status measures in different ethnic/racial groups with early rheumatoid arthritis: Implications for interpretation of clinical trial data. *J Rheumatol.* 2007;34:311–15.

[22] Margaretten M, Barton J, Julian L, et al. Socioeconomic determinants of disability and depression in patients with rheumatoid arthritis. *Arthritis Care Res.* 2011;63:24-246.

[23] Karpouzas GA, Dolatabadi S, Moran R, Li N, Nicassio M, & Wiseman MH. Correlates and predictors of disability in vulnerable US US Hispanics with rheumatoid arthritis. *Arthritis Care Res* (Hoboken) 2012;64:1274-81.

[24] McBurney CA, Vina ER. Racial and ethnic disparities in rheumatoid arthritis. *Current Rheumatology Reports.* 2012;14:463-71.

[25] Katz PP, Barton J, Trupin L, Schmajuk G, Yazdany J, Ruiz PJ, Yelin E. Poverty, Depression, or Lost in Translation? Ethnic and Language Variation in Patient-Reported Outcomes in Rheumatoid Arthritis. *Arthritis Care Res* (Hoboken) 2016, 68(5):621-8.

[26] Centers for Disease Control and Prevention. Racial/ethnic differences in the prevalence and impact of doctor-diagnosed arthritis— United States, 2002. *Morbidity and Mortality Weekly Report.* 2005;54, 119– 123.

[27] Katz PP, Yelin EH. Prevalence and correlates of depressive symptoms among persons with rheumatoid arthritis. *J Rheumatol.* 1993;20:790-796.

[28] Evers AWM, Kraaimaat FW, Geenen R, Jacobs JWG, Bijlsma JWJ. Long-term predictors of anxiety and depressed mood in early rheumatoid arthritis: A 3 and 5 year follow up. *J of Rheumatol.* 2002:29;2327-2336.

[29] Li X, Gignac MAM, Anis AH. The indirect costs of arthritis resulting from unemployment, reduced performance, and occupational changes while at work. *Medical Care.* 2006;44:304-310.

[30] Katz PP, Yelin EH. The development of depressive symptoms among women with rheumatoid-arthritis – The role of function. *Arthritis and Rheumatism.* 1995;38:49-56.

[31] Wolfe F. A reappraisal of HAQ disability in rheumatoid arthritis. *Arthritis and Rheumatism.* 2000;43:2751-61.

[32] Katz PP, Yelin EH. Activity loss and the onset of depressive symptoms – Do some activities matter more than others? *Arthritis and Rheumatism.* 2001;44:1194-1202.

[33] El-Miedany YM, El Rasheed AH. Is anxiety a more common disorder than depression in rheumatoid arthritis? *Joint Bone Spine* 2002;69:300-6.

[34] Cadena J, Vinaccia S, Perez A, Rico MI, Hinojosa R. The impact of disease activity on the quality of life, mental health status, and family dysfunction among Colombian patients with rheumatoid arthritis. *J of Clin Rheumatology*. 2003;9:142-150.

[35] Covic T, Adamson B, Spencer D, Howe G. A biopsychosocial model of pain and depression in rheumatoid arthritis: a 12-month longitudinal study. *Rheumatology*. 2003;42:1287-1294.

[36] Neugebauer A, Katz PP. Impact of social support on valued activity disability and depressive symptoms in patients with rheumatoid arthritis. *Arthritis Rheum*. 2004;51:586-92.

[37] Nakajima, A, Kamitsuji, S, Saito, A, Tanaka, E, Nishimura, K, Hoirikawa, N. et al. Disability and patient's appraisal of general health contribute to depressed mood in rheumatoid arthritis in a large clinical study in Japan. *Mod Rheumtaol*. 2006; 16:151-7.

[38] Katz, P., and Morris, A. Time use patterns among women with rheumatoid arthritis: Association with functional limitations and psychology status. *Rheumatology*. 2007;46.490-5.

[39] Smith BW, Zautra AJ. The effects of anxiety and depression on weekly pain in women with arthritis. *Pain*. 2008;138:354-61.

[40] Atal SA, Ceceli E, Okumu M et al. The evaluation of pain in patients with rheumatoid arthritis. *Pain Pract*. 2009;9:31.

[41] Van't Land H, Verdurmen J, Ten Have M, et al. The association between arthritis and psychiatric disorders; results from a longitudinal population-based study. *J Psychosom Res*. 2010, 68:187-193.

[42] Rezai F, Doost HTN, Molavi H, Abedi MR, Karimifar M. Depression and pain in patients with rheumatoid arthritis: Mediating role of illness perception. *The Egyptian Rheumatologist*. 2014;36:57-64.

[43] Benka J, Nagyova I, Rosenberger J, et al. Social participation in early and established rheumatoid arthritis patients. *Disability and Rehabilitation.* 2016;38:1172-79.

[44] Joyce AT, Smith P, Khandker R, Melin JM, Singh A. Hidden cost of rheumatoid arthritis (RA): Estimating cost of comorbid cardiovascular disease and depression among patients with RA. *J Rheumatol*. 2009;36:743-52.

[45] DiMatteo MR, Lepper HS, Croghan TW. Depression is a risk factor for noncompliance with medical treatment: meta-analysis of the effects of anxiety and depression on patient adherence. *Arch Intern Med.* 2000;160:2101-7.

[46] McNamara D, Stebbings S, Highton J. Severe osteoarthritis is associated with similar fatigue and greater pain scores than rheumatoid arthritis, at comparable levels of disability. *Rheumatology*. 2007:46;160.

[47] Julian LJ, Yelin E, Yazdany J, et al. Depression, medication adherence, and service utilization in systemic lupus erythematosus. *Arthritis Rheum.* 2009;61:240–246.

[48] Nicassio PM, Ormseth SR, Kay M, et al. The contribution of pain and depression to self-reported sleep disturbance in patients with rheumatoid arthritis. *Pain,* 2012, 153:107-12.

[49] Katz, P. Causes and consequences of fatigue in rheumatoid arthritis. *Curr Opin Rheumatol* 2017;29:269-276.

[50] Scherrer JF, Virgo KS, Zeringue A, et al. Depression increases risk of incident myocardial infarction among veterans administration patients with rheumatoid arthritis. *Gen Hosp Psych* 2009;31:353-9.

[51] Fuller-Thomson E, Shaked Y. Factors associated with depression and suicidal ideation among individuals with arthritis or rheumatism: findings from a representative community survey. *Arthritis Rhe*um. 2009; 61:944–50.

[52] Treharne GJ, Lyons AC, Kitas GD. Suicidal ideation in patients with rheumatoid arthritis: research may help identify patients at high risk. *BMJ.* 2000; 321:1290.

[53] Pincus T. Is mortality increased in patients with rheumatoid arthritis? *J Musculoskeletal Med.* 1988; 5:27–46.

[54] Ang, DC. Choi, H., Kroenke, K., Wolfe, F. Comorbid depression is an independent risk factor for mortality in patients with rheumatoid arthritis. *J Rheumatol.* 2005;32:1013-1019.

[55] Fuller-Thomson E, Shaked Y. Factors associated with depression and suicidal ideation among individuals with arthritis or rheumatism: Findings from a representative community survey. *Arthritis Rheum.* 2009;61:944-950.

[56] Nicassio PM. The problem of detecting and managing depression in the rheumatology clinic. *Arthritis Care Res.* 2008, 59:155-158.

[57] Roubille C, Richer V, Starnino T, et al. Evidence-based recommendations for the management of comorbidities in rheumatoid arthritis, psoriasis, and psoriatic arthritis: Expert opinion of the Canadian Dermatology-Rheumatology Comorbidity Initiative. *J Rheumatol.* 2015;42:1767-80.

[58] Plach SK, Napholz L, Kelber ST. Social, health, and age differences associated with depressive disorders in women with rheumatoid arthritis. *Int J Aging Human Dev.* 2005:61;179-194.

[59] Doeglas, DM., Suurmeijer, TPBM., van den Heuvel, WJA, et al. Functional ability, social support, and depression in rheumatoid arthritis. *Quality of Life Research*. 2004;13:1053-1065.

[60] Katz PP, Neugebauer A. Does satisfaction with abilities mediate the relationship between the impact of rheumatoid arthritis on valued activities and depressive symptoms? *Arthritis Rheum.* 2001;45:263-269.

[61] Neugebauer A, Katz PP, Pasch LA. Effect of valued activity disability, social comparisons, and satisfaction with ability on depressive symptoms in rheumatoid arthritis. *Health Psychol.* 2003;22(3):253-62.

[62] Karpouzas GA, Draper T, Moran R, Hernandez E, Nicassio P, Weisman MH, Ormseth S. Trends in Functional Disability and Determinants of Clinically Meaningful Change Over Time in

Hispanic Patients With Rheumatoid Arthritis in the US. *Arthritis Care Res* (Hoboken). 2017;69(2):294-298.

[63] Bazzichi L, Maser J, Piccinni A, et al. Quality of life in rheumatoid arthritis: Impact of disability and lifetime depressive spectrum symptomatology. *Clinical and Experimental Rheumatology.* 2005;23:783-788.

[64] Piccini A, Maser JD, Bazzichi L, et al. Clinical significance of lifetime mood and panic-agoraphobic spectrum symptoms on quality of life of patients with rheumatoid arthritis. *Comprehensive Psychiatry.* 2006;47:201-208.

[65] Ormseth SR, Draper TL, Irwin MR, et al. A multidimensional model of disability and role functioning in rheumatoid arthritis. *Arthritis Care Res.* 2015;67(12):1686-92.

[66] Michaud K, Wolfe F. Comorbidities in rheumatoid arthritis. *Best Practices Res Clin Rheumatol.* 2007;21:885-906.

[67] Béland Y. Canadian community health survey--methodological overview. *Health Rep.* 2002;13(3):9-14.

[68] Pinto-Gouveia J, Costa J, Maroco J. The first 2-years of rheumatoid arthritis: The influence of acceptance on pain, physical limitation and depression. *J Health Psychol.* 2013;20:102-112.

[69] Linton, SJ, Nicholas MK, MacDonald S, Boersma K, Bergbom S, Maher C, Refshauge K. The role of depression and catastrophizing in musculoskeletal pain. *Eur J Pain.* 2011, 15(4):416-22.

[70] Edwards RR, Bingham CO, Bathon J, Haythornthwaite JA. Catastrophizing and pain in arthritis, fibromyalgia, and other rheumatic diseases. *Arthritis Rheum* 2006;55:325–332.

[71] Evers AW, Verhoeven EW, van Middendorp H, et al. Does Stress affect the joints? Daily stressors, stress vulnerability, immune and HPA axis activity, and short-term disease and symptoms fluctuation in rheumatoid arthritis. *Ann Rheum Dis.* 2014;73:1683-8.

[72] Edwards RR, Cahalan C, Mensing G, Smith M, Haythornthwaite JA. Pain, catastrophizing, and depression in rheumatic diseases. *Nature Reviews Rheumatology.* 2011;7:216-224.

[73] Treharne GJ, Kitas GD, Lyons AC, Booth DA. Well-being in rheumatoid arthritis: the effects of disease duration and psychosocial factors. *J Health Psychol*. 2005;10(3):457-74.

[74] Dowdy SW, Dwyer KA, Smith CA, Wallston KA. Gender and psychological well-being of persons with rheumatoid arthritis. *Arthritis Care and Research.* 1996;9:449-456.

[75] Theis KA, Hootman JM, Helmick GG, et al. State-specific prevalence of arthritis-attributable work limitation – United States, 2003 (Reprinted from MMWR, vol 56, pg 1045-1049,2007). *JAMA*. 2007;298:2255-225.

[76] Jacob L, Rockel T, Kostev K. *Depression risk in patients with rheumatoid arthritis in the United Kingdom 2017*. Accessed 29 April 2007 at: http://www.medengine.com/Redeem/C3F7F0602F1 29F4E (29).

[77] Fisher L, Chesla CA, Mullan JT, Skaff MM, Kanter RA. Contributors to depression in Latino and European-American patients with type 2 diabetes. *Diabetes Care.* 2001;24(10):1751-7.

[78] Wright SJ, Barnard MU, Olson NY, Austin JS, Lindsley CB. Communication issues of young adults with arthritis. *Arthritis and Rheumatism.* 1998;41:S250.

[79] Packham JC, Hall MA, Pimm TJ. Long-term follow-up of 246 adults with juvenile idiopathic arthritis: predictive factors for mood and pain. *Rheumatology*. 2002;41:1444-1449.

[80] Harrison MJ, Farragher TM, Clarke AM, Manning SC, Bunn DK, Symmons DP. Association of functional outcome with both personal and area-level socioeconomic inequalities in patients with inflammatory polyarthritis. *Arthritis Rheum*. 2009;61:1297–304.

[81] Patten SB, Williams JV, Lavorato DH, et al. Patterns of association of chronic medical conditions and major depression. *Epidemiol Psychiatr Sci.* 2016, 27:1-9.

[82] Sleath B, Chewning B, de Vellis BM, et al. Communication about depression during rheumatoid arthritis patient visits. *Arthritis Rheum* 2008;15:186-191.

[83] Nicassio, PM, Irani, M. Depression in Rheumatoid Arthritis. *The Rheumatologist* 2012. Accessed 29 April 2017 at: http://www.the-rheumatologist.org/article/depression-in-rheumatoid-arthritis/4/

[84] Sleath B, Rubin RH. Gender, ethnicity, and physician-patient communication about depression and anxiety in primary care. *Patient Educ Couns.* 2002;48(3):243-52.

[85] Fiest KM, Hitchon CA, Bernstein CN, et al. Defining the Burden and Managing the Effects of Psychiatric Comorbidity in Chronic Immunoinflammatory Disease. Systematic Review and Meta-analysis of Interventions for Depression and Anxiety in Persons with Rheumatoid Arthritis. *J Clin Rheumatol.* 2017.

[86] Hayes S. Acceptance and commitment therapy, relational frame theory, and the third wave of behavioral and cognitive therapies. *Behavior Therapy*. 2004;35: 639–665.

[87] Vowles K, McCracken L, Eccleston C. (2008) Patient functioning and catastrophizing in chronic pain: The mediating effects of acceptance. *Health Psychology*. 2008;27(2 Suppl.): S136–S143.

[88] McCracken L, Vowles K. A prospective analysis of acceptance of pain and values-based action in patients with chronic pain. *Health Psychology*. 2008;27: 215–220.

[89] Singh N, Lancioni G, Wahler R, et al. Mindfulness approaches in cognitive behavior therapy. *Behavioural and Cognitive Psychotherapy*. 2008;36: 659–666.

[90] Viane I, Crombez G, Eccleston C, et al. Acceptance of pain is an independent predictor of mental well-being in patients with chronic pain: Empirical evidence and reappraisal. *Pain.* 2003;106: 65–72.

[91] McCracken L. *Contextual Cognitive Behavioral Therapy for Chronic Pain* 2005;33. Seattle, WA: IASP Press.

[92] McCracken L, Gauntlett-Gilbert J, Vowles K. The role of mindfulness in a contextual cognitive analysis of chronic pain-related suffering and disability. *Pain.* 2007;131: 63–69.

[93] Nicholas M and Asghari A (2006) Investigating acceptance in adjustment to chronic pain: Is acceptance broader than we thought? *Pain.* 124: 269–279.

[94] Kollman D, Brown T, Barlow D. The construct validity of acceptance: A multitrait-multimethod investigation. *Behavior Therapy*. 2009;40: 205–218.

[95] Garfenski N, Kraaij V, Benoist M, Bout Z, Karels E, Smit A. Effect of a cognitive behavioral self-help intervention on depression, anxiety, and coping self-efficacy in people with rheumatic disease. *Arthritis Care Res.* 2013;65:1077-1084.

[96] Pradhan E, Baumgarten M, Langenberg P, et al. Effect of mindfulness-based stress reduction in rheumatoid arthritis patients. *Arthritis Rheum.* 2007;57:1134-42.

[97] Zautra AJ, Davis MC, Reich JW, et al. Comparison of cognitive behavioral and mindfulness meditation interventions on adaptation to rheumatoid arthritis for patients with and without history of recurrent depression. *J Consult Clin Psychol*. 2008;76:408-21.

[98] Neuberger GB, Aaronson LS, Gajewski B, et al. Predictors of exercise and effects of exercise on symptoms, function, aerobic fitness, and disease outcomes of rheumatoid arthritis. *Arthritis and Rheumatism (Arthritis Care and Research)* 2007;57(6);943-52.

[99] Herring MP, Puetz TW, O'connor PJ, Dishman RK. Effects of exercise training on depressive symptoms among patients with a chronic illness: A systematic review and meta-analysis of randomized controlled trials. *Arch Int Med.* 2012;172:101-111.

[100] Cooney G, Dwan K, Greig C, Lawlor D, Rimer J, Waugh F, McMurdo M, Mead B. Exercise for depression. Cochrane Database Syst Rev. 2013; 9. Art. No CD004366. Kelley GA, Kelley KS, Hootman JM. Effects of exercise on depression in adults with arthritis: A systematic review with meta-analysis of randomized controlled trials. *Arthritis Research and Therapy* 2015;17(1):21.

[101] Middleton KR, Ward MM, Haaz S, Velummylum S, Fike A, Acevedo AT, Tataw-Ayuketah G, Dietz L, Mittleman BB, Wallen GR. A pilot study of yoga as self-care for arthritis in minority communities. *Health Qual Life Outcomes*. 2013;2;11:55.

[102] Ishikawa RZ, Cardemil EV, Falmagne RJ. Help seeking and help receiving for emotional distress among Latino men and women. *Qual Health Res.* 2010;20(11):1558-72.

[103] Bell RA, Franks P, Duberstein PR, Epstein RM, Feldman MD, Fernandez y Garcia E, Kravitz RL. Suffering in silence: reasons for not disclosing depression in primary care. *Ann Fam Med.* 2011;9(5):439-46.

[104] Hansen MC, Cabassa LJ. Pathways to depression care: help-seeking experiences of low-income Latinos with diabetes and depression. *J Immigr Minor Health.* 2012;14(6):1097-106.

[105] Hansen MC, Cabassa LJ. Pathways to depression care: help-seeking experiences of low-income Latinos with diabetes and depression. *J Immigr Minor Health.* 2012;14(6):1097-106.

[106] Cabassa LJ, Hansen MC, Palinkas LA, Ell K. Azúcar y nervios: explanatory models and treatment experiences of Hispanics with diabetes and depression. *Soc Sci Med.* 2008 Jun;66(12):2413-24.

[107] Cabassa LJ, Lester R, Zayas LH. "It's like being in a labyrinth:" Hispanic immigrants' perceptions of depression and attitudes toward treatments. *J Immigr Minor Health*. 2007;9(1):1-16.

[108] Givens JL, Houston TK, Van Voorhees BW, Ford DE, Cooper LA. Ethnicity and preferences for depression treatment. *Gen Hosp Psychiatry.* 2007;29(3):182-91.

[109] Interian A, Martinez IE, Guarnaccia PJ, Vega WA, Escobar JI. A qualitative analysis of the perception of stigma among Latinos receiving antidepressants. *Psychiatr Serv.* 2007;58:1591–4.

[110] Cooper LA, Gonzales JJ, Gallo JJ, Rost KM, Meredith LS, Rubenstein LV, Wang NY, Ford DE. The acceptability of treatment for depression among African-American, Hispanic, and white primary care patients. *Med Care*. 2003;41(4):479-89.

[111] Dwight-Johnson M, Sherbourne CD, Liao D, Wells KB. Treatment preferences among depressed primary care patients. *J Gen Intern Med.* 2000;15(8):527-34.

[112] Dwight-Johnson M, Lagomasino IT, Aisenberg E, Hay J. Using conjoint analysis to assess depression treatment preferences among low-income Latinos. *Psychiatr Serv.* 2004;55(8):934-6.

[113] Karasz A, Watkins L. Conceptual models of treatment in depressed Hispanic patients. *Ann Fam Med.* 2006;4(6):527-33.

[114] Berrios-Rivera JP, Street Jr RL, Garcia Popa-Lisseanu MG, et al. Trust in physicians and elements of the medical interaction in patients with rheumatoid arthritis and systemic lupus erythematosus. *Arthritis Rheum.* 2006;55:385–93.

[115] Vega WA, Rodriguez MA, Ang A. Addressing stigma of depression in Latino primary care patients. *Gen Hosp Psychiatr.* 2010; 32:182–91.

[116] Caplan S, Escobar J, Paris M, Alvidrez J, Dixon JK, Desai MM, Scahill LD, Whittemore R. Cultural influences on causal beliefs about depression among Latino immigrants. *J Transcult Nurs.* 2013;24(1):68-77.

[117] Añez LM, Paris M Jr, Bedregal LE, Davidson L, Grilo CM. Application of cultural constructs in the care of first generation Latino clients in a community mental health setting. *J Psychiatr Pract.* 2005;11(4):221-30.

[118] Chong J, Reinschmidt KM, Moreno FA. Symptoms of depression in a Hispanic primary care population with and without chronic medical illnesses. *Prim Care Companion J Clin Psychiatry.* 2010;12(3).

[119] Interian A, Martinez IE, Guarnaccia PJ, Vega WA, Escobar JI. A qualitative analysis of the perception of stigma among Latinos receiving antidepressants. *Psychiatr Serv.* 2007; 58:1591–4.

[120] 121.Nadeem E, Lange JM, Edge D, Fongwa M, Belin T, Miranda J. Does stigma keep poor young immigrant and U.S.-born Black and Latina women from seeking mental health care? *Psychiatr Serv.* 2007; 58(12):1547–54.

[121] Pincay, IEM, Guarnaccia, PJ. ''It's like going through an earthquake'': anthropological perspectives on depression among Latino immigrants. *Journal of Immigrant Health* 2007;9, 17–28.

[122] Perez MC and Fortuna L. Psychosocial stressors, psychiatric diagnosis, and utilization of mental health services among undocumented immigrant Latinos. *Journal of Immigrant & Refugee Services.* 2005;3, 107-123.

[123] Lackey GF. "Feeling blue" in Spanish: a qualitative inquiry of depression among Mexican immigrants. *Soc Sci Med.* 2008;67(2):228-37.

[124] Callahan LF, Cleveland RJ, Li X, et al. Current social position associated with rheumatoid arthritis severity and self-reported health outcomes in African Americans. *Arthritis Rheum.* 2011;63 Suppl 10:1545.

[125] Cleveland RJ, Schwartz TA, Jonas BL, et al. Influence of lifecourse social position on rheumatoid arthritis disease severity in African Americans. *Arthritis Rheum.* 2011;63 Suppl 10:2642.

[126] Karasz A. Cultural differences in conceptual models of depression. *Soc Sci Med.* 2005; 60:1625– 1635.

[127] Bruce B, Fries JF. Rheumatologist perceptions of sources of health care disparities in minority rheumatoid arthritis patients. *J Clin Rheumatol.* 2009;15:145–7.

[128] McIlvane JM. Disentangling the effects of race and SES on arthritis-related symptoms, coping, and well-being in African American and White women. *Aging Ment Health.* 2007;11(5):556-69.

[129] McIlvane JM, Baker TA, Mingo CA. Racial differences in arthritis-related stress, chronic life stress, and depressive symptoms among women with arthritis: a contextual perspective. *J Gerontol B Psychol Sci Soc Sci.* 2008;63(5):S320-7.

[130] Barton JL, Trupin L, Schillinger D, et al. Racial and ethnic disparities in disease activity and function among persons with rheumatoid arthritis from university-affiliated clinics. *Arthritis Care Res* (Hoboken). 2011;63:1238–46.

[131] Suarez-Almazor ME, Berrios-Rivera JP, Cox V, Janssen NM, Marcus DM, Sessoms S. Initiation of disease-modifying

antirheumatic drug therapy in minority and disadvantaged patients with rheumatoid arthritis. *J Rheumatol.* 2007;34:2400–7.

[132] Garcia-Gonzalez A, Richardson M, Garcia Popa-Lisseanu M, et al. Treatment adherence in patients with rheumatoid arthritis and systemic lupus erythematosus. *Clin Rheumatol*. 2008;27:883–9.

[133] Cannon GW, Mikuls TR, Hayden CL, et al. Merging Veterans Affairs rheumatoid arthritis registry and pharmacy data to assess methotrexate adherence and disease activity in clinical practice. *Arthritis Care Res* (Hoboken). 2011;63:1680–90.

## Biographical Sketch

### *Mellissa Withers*

**Affiliation:**

Associate Professor, University of Southern California, Keck School of Medicine, Department of Preventive Medicine

**Education:**

*University of California at Los Angeles*-Los Angeles, California

Ph.D. - Fielding School of Public Health, Community Health Sciences Department.

*Johns Hopkins Bloomberg School of Public Health* - Baltimore, Maryland

Master of Health Science - International Health, Health Systems Management track.

*University of California at Berkeley*- Berkeley, California

B. A. - Global Development Studies.

**Business Address:**

2001 N Soto Street, SSB 318G, Los Angeles, CA 90089 USA

**Research and Professional Experience:**

Dr. Mellissa Withers is an Associate Professor at the University of Southern California Keck School of Medicine in the Institute for Global Health. She also leads the Global Health Program of the Association of Pacific Rim Universities, a network of 50 universities in the Pacific Rim region. She has conducted numerous studies relating to immigrants, including intimate partner violence among immigrant women, human trafficking in Los Angeles, participation in cancer clinical trials among Latino immigrants, depression among Latinos in Los Angeles, genetic testing among families at risk for autosomal dominant Alzheimer's Disease, Mexican immigrant men's perspectives regarding family planning, and needs assessment of immigrants in Santiago, Chile using photovoice methodology. Her other research interests include: community participatory research, women's empowerment, human trafficking, gender-based violence, and global reproductive health. She teaches courses in global health, ethics, and leadership.

**Professional Appointments:**

University of Southern California, Institute for Global Health, School of Medicine- Los Angeles, California
Associate Professor, January 2013- present

Association of Pacific Rim Universities- Hong Kong
Director, Global Health Program, January 2013-present.

**Publications from the Last 3 Years:**

Choudhury, S. M., Toller Erasquin, J., and Withers, M. (editors) *Global Perspectives on Women's Sexual and Reproductive Health Across the Lifespan.* Springer Publishers, 2017.

Withers, M, and Browner, C. (2017) "The role of Balinese culture in explaining inconsistencies between fertility intentions and reproductive outcomes." Choudhury, SM, Toller Erasquin, J., and Withers, M. (editors) *Global Perspectives on Women's Sexual and Reproductive Health Across the Lifespan.* Springer Publishers.

Withers, M, Li, M, Manalo, G, So, S, Wipfli, H, Khoo, HE, Wu, JTS, Lin, HH. (2017) "Best Practices in Global Health Practicums: Recommendations from the Association of Pacific Rim Universities." *Journal of Community Health*, e-published ahead of print.

Withers, M, Kharazmi, N, Lim, E. (2017) "Traditional beliefs and practices during pregnancy, childbirth, and the post-partum period in Asian countries.' *Midwifery*, e-published ahead of print.

Wu, CF, Woodward, A, Li, Y, Kan, H, Balasubramanian, R, Latif, MT, Sahani, M, Cheng, TJ, Chio, Cp, Taneepanichskul, N, Kim, H, Chan, CC, Yi, SM, Withers, M, Samet, J. (2017) "Regulation of Fine Particulate Matter ($PM_{2.5}$) in the Pacific Rim: Perspectives from the APRU Global Health Program." *Air Quality, Atmosphere & Health,* in press.

Withers, M, Gonzalez, L, Karpouzas, G. (2017) "Identification and Treatment Optimization of Co-morbid Depression in Rheumatoid Arthritis." *Rheumatology and Therapy*, 4(2):281-291.

Tuan, NT, Withers, M, Hajeebhoy, N, Frongillo, EA. (2016) "Estimates of the quality of complementary feeding among Vietnamese infants aged 6−23 months varied by how commercial baby cereals were classified in 24-hour recalls." *Maternal and Child Nutrition*, e-published ahead of print,

Prata, N, Fraser, A. Huchko, MJ, Gipson, JD, Withers, M, Lewis, S, Ciaraldi, EJ, Upadhyay, UD. (2016) "Women's Empowerment and Family Planning: A Review of the Literature." *Journal of Biosocial Sciences*, 10:1-31, 2017.

Samet J. and Withers, M. (2016) "The APRU Global Health Program: Past and Future." *Journal of Epidemiology*, 26(4): 166-170.

Tuan, NT, Withers, M, Hajeebhoy, N, Frongillo, EA. (2016) "Feeding of infant formula at birth is common and associated with subsequent breastfeeding behavior: a representative study from Vietnam." *Journal of Nutrition.* 146(10):2102-2108, Epub 2016 Sep 7.

Withers, M, Press, D, Wipfli, H, McCool, J, Chan, CC, Jimba, M, Tremewan, C, Samet, J. (2016) "Training the next generation of global health experts: experiences and recommendations from Pacific Rim universities." *Globalization and Health,* 12(1): 34.

Tavrow, P, Bloom, B, Withers, M. (2016) Intimate partner violence screening practices in California after passage of the Affordable Care Act. *Violence Against Women*, e-published ahead of print.

Harrington, E, Dworkin, S, Withers, M and Newmann, S. (2016) "Gendered power dynamics and women's negotiation of family planning in the context of HIV: A qualitative study of couples in western Kenya." *Culture, Health and Sexuality*, 18(4):453-69.

Browner, C. and Withers, M. (2015) "Reproduction" *Encyclopedia of Human Sexuality,* Eds. Patricia Wheelan and Anne Bolin, Wiley-Blackwell, Hoboken, New Jersey.

Withers, M., Dworkin, S., Zakaras, J. M., Onono, M., Oyier, B, Cohen, C., Bukusi, E. and Newmann, S. (2015) "Women Now Wear Trousers": Men's Perceptions of Family Planning Use in the Context of Changing Gender Relations in Western Kenya." *Culture, Health and Sexuality, 17(9): 1132-1146.*

Withers, M., Dworkin, S., Onono, M., Oyier, B, Grossman, D., Cohen, C., Bukusi, E. and Newmann, S. (2015) How should men's involvement in family planning be increased? A view of men's perspectives in Nyanza Province, Kenya. *Studies in Family Planning,* 46(2): 201-215.

Furthermore, presence of inflammatory joint signs in a cohort of RA first-degree relatives at baseline and at 2 years was significantly associated with smoking >10 pack-years compared to never smokers. First degree relatives younger than 50 years with >10 pack-years had the highest risk of inflammatory joint sign (OR 4.39. 95% CI 2.22-8.66) compared to never smokers and younger age [26]. Not only, among asymptomatic RA first-degree relatives, current smoking and smoking >10 pack-years were associated with two-fold increased risk of developing inflammatory arthritis [26].

Even the snuff (smokeless tobacco), prepared from dried tobacco leaves, carries the risk of exposure to nicotine with the levels of blood and urine nicotine/cotinine being comparable to those of smokers [27, 28]. Limited studies, however they are somewhat limited, reported no association between usage of snuff and risk of development of RA (regardless of autoantibodies) [29, 30]. In the strength of these findings, Jiang et al. reported that smoking increased risk of RA is most probably not due to nicotine, given that the use of smokeless tobacco containing nicotine was not associated with the risk of RA, regardless of autoantibodies status [29]. Future studies concerning smoking status in RA should focus on different smoke status and/or products.

## Gender-Difference in the Susceptibility of Smoking to RA

Cigarette smoking was reported to be gender-specific in its ability to trigger the development of RA [15]. However, the findings were contradictory as some studies demonstrated that smoking increases the risk of RA in women [13, 31]. In a meta-analysis reviewing this association, the risk for female smokers to develop RA was 1.3 times greater than that of non-smokers [13]. While other reports did not confirm this association in women [15, 32]. In contrast, it has been reported that the risk of RA was significantly higher in men than in women [15], and the risk for smokers is about twice that of male non-smokers [13].

## Smoking-Genetic Interaction in the Susceptibility of RA Development

It is well known that the gene-environment interaction between smoking and HLA-DRB1 shared epitope (SE) genotype remarkably increase the risk of RA [7], in particular with seropositive cases [14, 33]. The study among Asian RA populations showed an interaction between smoking and SE carriage influencing the risk and pathogenesis of RA, however, these findings were not strong as reported in European or North American RA patients [25].

The association of polymorphism of the PTPN22 gene with smoking increases the risk of anti-cyclic citrullinated peptide antibody (ACPA) positivity RA [34]. However, no interaction between smoking status and PTPN22 R620W for either ACPA positive or negative RA patients was found [35]. These findings may add strength to the previous finding of SE-smoking interaction, since this interaction is shown to be specific to SE and not seen in other genes related to RA risk and pathogenesis (e.g., PTPN22) [36].

Gene p53 overexpression in carcinomas of lung, upper airway and bladder was observed to be related to smoking exposure [37]. Studies examining the pathogenesis of RA joint inflammation led to the demonstration that the p53 tumor suppressor gene is overexpressed in RA synovium and in fibroblast-like synoviocytes [38, 39]. Sun et al., pointed that there are number of inflammatory cytokines believed to play a role in the pathogenesis of RA, such as interleukin (IL)-6, that is upregulated by p53 gene [40].

The search for new genes which predispose to RA risk is continuous, thus the search for gene–environment interactions such as smoking should keep in parallel.

## Smoking Intensity and Risk of RA Development

Previous epidemiological studies showed an increasing risk of developing RA with the intensity (pack-years) and the duration of smoking [11, 31, 41]; however, a meta-analysis showed that even light smoking had a connection with the development of RA [12].

The risk of developing RA from gene–environment interactions is not restricted to the smoking exposure but also increases with its intensity. Having an SE and a smoking dose more than 20 packs/year were independent risk factors for the development of RA with a high tier of ACPA [42]. In the Nurses' Health Study, there is evidence of multiplicative smoking-SE interaction with the highest risk of seropositive RA in heavy smokers who carry two copies of the SE [43].

## Smoking Screening for the Development of RA

Screening for RA implicates the identification of asymptomatic patients, at very early stage of the disease, assuming that prevention strategies; however, they are not available up to date, can be applied [40]. Variables which have been identified for screening of preclinical RA includes genetic, serological and environmental factors. RA prediction models based on genetic variants and smoking status exist and potentially play a role in screening the general population with a family history of RA [21]. Identifying modifiable risk factors such as smoking, periodontitis, obesity, viral infections, hormonal and dietary factors will be useful in preventing RA in susceptible populations [36].

# Impact of Smoking on RA Immunity

Chronic cigarette smoking act on both innate and adaptive immune system to produce a systemic pro-inflammatory state [44].

## Cigarette Smoke and Innate Immunity

Lungs are an important path of exposure to environmental pathogens and antigens. Immune defense mechanisms, via alveolar macrophages (AMs) and other monocytes, are involved in the innate immune response in the lungs [44]. However, cigarette smoking increases the number of AMs by several fold [45], AMs from smokers have a reduced function; for example their ability to phagocytose and/or kill bacteria. It has been reported that AMs from smokers secrete significantly lower levels of pro-inflammatory cytokines [46].

## Cigarette Smoke and Adaptive Immunity

### *Humeral Immunity*

The negative effects of smoking on the humoral immune response have been studied and considered as one of the master mechanisms linking smoking with chronic autoimmune disease as RA [47].

Extensive data suggest that smoking modulate the immune system and are contributing to a shift from T helper (Th)-1 to Th-2 immune response. RA-associated pro-inflammatory cytokines/chemokines, such as tumor necrosis factor (TNF)-α, IL-1, IL-6, IL-8, IL-13 and granulocyte-macrophage colony-stimulating factor (GM-CSF) were significantly higher in current smokers compared with former or never smokers [44, 48–52]. It is well known that TNF-α, IL-1 and IL-6 have been remarkably contributing in the pathogenesis of RA [46]. Furthermore, smoking induces increase levels of Th-17 cells and its pro-inflammatory cytokines IL-17 [53]. Recently, Th-17 and IL-17 have shown to be contributor to RA pathogenesis [54]. Receptor activator of nuclear factor kappa-B ligand (RANKL) and osteoprotegerin (OPG) are important cytokines in the pathogenesis and joints erosion of RA [46, 55]. Smokers have shown to increase RANKL/OPG ratio in serum [56]. Cigarette smoking increased the expression of matrix metalloproteinase (MMP)-12, which is produced by both macrophages and dendritic cells in the lungs of mice [57]. MMP-

12 has been involved in the pathogenesis of RA [58] and particularly in RA synovial tissues and consequence cartilage damage [58]. Moreover, smokers show high levels of pro MMP-9 [59], derived from RA synovial fibroblasts, and involved in articular cartilage destruction [60]. Smoking increases the levels of several inflammatory indices, including C-reactive protein (CRP) [61]. Autoantibodies levels such as anti-nuclear are higher among smokers with autoimmune diseases like RA [44, 62–65]. Smoking exposure, in particular nicotine, can increase the oxidative stress through increasing both endogenous and exogenous free radicals in the body [66], which have a role in the pathogenesis of RA [67].

On the other hand, smoking had suppressive effect on IL-6 production through Toll-like receptors (TLR)-2 and 9, decreased IL-10 production via TLR-2 activation. Through mononuclear cells, smoking also decreased production of IL-1b, IL-2, TNF-α, and interferon (IFN)-γ [68, 69]. The inhibitory effects of cigarette smoking have been attributed to nicotine, hydroquinone and to carbon monoxide in the smoke. Thus, nicotine inhibits endothelial cell release of IL-8, a potent leukocyte chemotactic factor, specific for neutrophils [70]. Yu et al. showed that nicotine pretreatment aggravated the disease in rat model of RA, while nicotine post-treatment suppressed the disease [71]. The mixed effect of smoking on immune system is demonstrated on Figure 1.

### *Cellular Immunity*

Chronic smoke exposure, especially with long duration, is associated with decrease leucocyte function and serum immunoglobulin [44, 72].

Neutrophils are the most frequent type of leukocytes and play a major role in the body defense against bacterial invasion [73]. Nicotine-induced secretion of catecholamines, increases the peripheral polymorphonuclear neutrophils (PMN) counts, inhibit formation of free oxygen radicals in PMN and reduce their function. Smokers-PMN show depressed migration and chemotaxis compared with non-smokers PMN [74]. However, smokers have a higher number of circulating PMNs compared with non-smokers, it is likely that nicotine suppresses PMNs inflammatory mediated mechanisms [48].

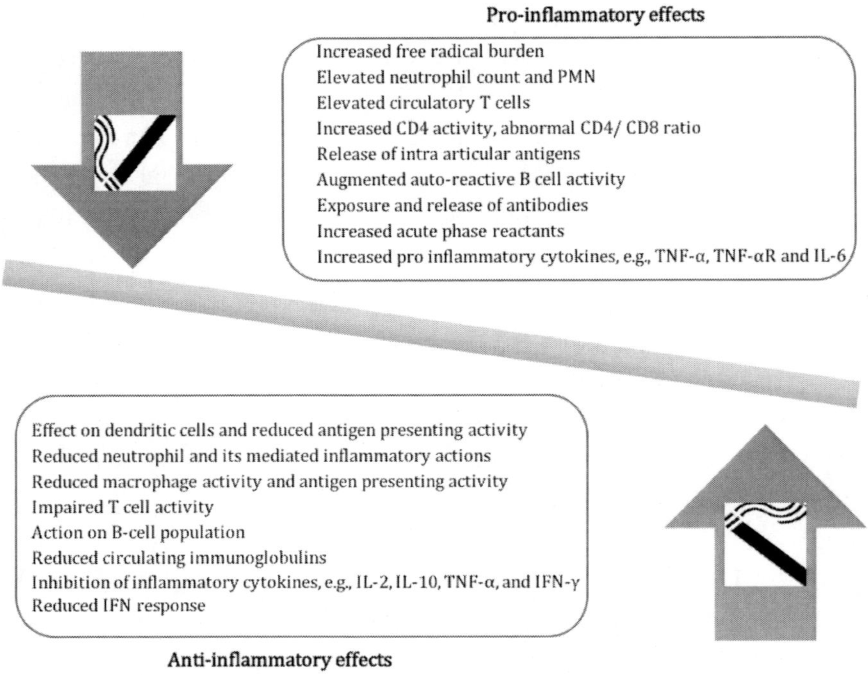


Figure 1. Paradoxical effects (pro-inflammatory and anti-inflammatory) of cigarette smoking exposure on the function of immune system.

Resident alveolar macrophages, the main lung cells, serve as the first line of cellular defense against toxins due to their antigen-presenting function and phagocytic properties. Smoke particles (mainly kaolinit) are detected in the cytoplasm of alveolar macrophages [8]. Natural killer (NK) cells are reduced in smokers and previous reports suggest that NK cells have both protective and detrimental roles in RA [75]. Nicotine contributes to autoimmunity by maintaining the non-exhausted phenotype of $CD8^{+}$T cells resulting in the release of survivin. Survivin is an inhibitor of apoptosis, that can be measured in serum of RA patients to predict poor disease outcome and poor response to therapy [76].

Fibroblast-like synoviocytes (FLS), the thin layer of cells of the synovial membrane, secrete a protein involved in joint lubrication called lubricin [77, 78]. Synovial hyperplasia and proliferation of FLS into several layers are characteristics features of RA. In RA, FLS secrete pro-inflammatory cytokines (IL-1, IL-6) MMP-9 and chemokines, which create local inflammatory status and add in joint destruction [77, 78]. Cigarette smoke induces pro-inflammatory cytokines in RA affected FLS [79]. Heat shock proteins (HSP), stress proteins, are shown to present in different stressful conditions, such as in RA due to the hypoxia induced by proliferated FLS [80]. Heat shock proteins are upregulated in the synovial tissues of smokers with RA, in contrast to non-smokers. In addition, HSP have been reported to increase the production of inflammatory cytokines and of matrix-degrading molecules via stimulating FLS [80].

### *Apoptosis*

Smoking has paradoxical effect on apoptosis, depending on the cell types [81, 82]. It can stimulate apoptosis via increase the percentage of Fas (CD96) and $CD4^{+}$T-cells that lead to high levels of cellular debris [81]. On the controversy, the soluble Fas levels were not higher in the saliva of smokers' than in that of non-smokers', suggesting that smoking might promote anti-apoptotic mechanisms in the oral cavity [83]. Also, Bijl et al. reported that Fas-induced apoptosis and the percentages of circulating apoptotic lymphocytes in vitro did not show differences between smokers and non-smokers [81]. These conflicting results of the effects of smoking on apoptosis necessitate further researching.

### *Epigenetic Modifications*

Smoking could lead to epigenetic changes such as DNA methylation [84]. DNA methylation appears to play crucial roles in gene modulation and increase risk of development of RA in susceptible individuals. The increased risk of RA associated with smoking might be mediated by epigenetic modifications, as smoking was significantly associated with hypomethylation of specific DNA regions [85].

# Association of Smoking with Clinical Manifestations, Serological Parameters and Therapeutic Response

## Clinical Manifestations

### *Articular*

Increased disease activity among current smokers was observed for nearly all components of the 28 joints disease activity score (DAS28), including tender and swollen joint counts and patient global assessment, although there was no association with erythrocytes sedimentation rate (ESR) [52]. Among ACPA positive patients, current smokers exhibited significantly higher levels of RA disease activity than never smokers. Also, former smokers demonstrated significantly lower levels of RA disease activity than current smokers [52]. In established RA, several studies confirmed that the disease activity score was higher in current and former smokers compared to never smokers [86–89].

In the Quintana-Dunque et al. [90] study of 129 early onset RA patients, they found that the baseline smoking status (ever vs. never; current vs. never) was inversely associated with disease activity and disability at 36 months. Not only with disease activity, cigarette smoking was associated with increased disease severity in early RA [91]. Moreover, in an early RA cohort, current smoking status was associated with a 4-fold higher risk for not achieving an American College of Rheumatology 50 response after adjustment for cofounders [92]. Several studies have cited smoking as a poor predictor of remission in patients with RA [93–95]. Inoue et al. [94] showed that the male patients in each smoking status (past and current compared to never smoking) were more likely to have lower disease activity scores in all the composite measures than female patients, and male never smokers tended to show higher remission proportions than past and current male smokers. The effects of smoking on remission remained different in relation to gender after multivariate analysis.

Controversy, studies showed that smoking may not be as detrimental as previously considered in RA disease course. In line with another multinational study [96], Krol et al. [97] found that disease activity was not associated with smoking status.

In comparison to active smoking, the effect of passive smoking (second-hand smoking), defined as the involuntary inhalation of tobacco smoking, on RA disease status has not been extensively studied. Passive smoking has been widely associated with several diseases, including cardiovascular diseases [46]. In a previous recent work, it was found that not only active smoking but also second-hand smoking has an impact on disease activity in women with RA [98].

***Extra-Articular***

The incidence of extra-articular manifestations (EAM) of RA is about 20%–45% [99–102], and it is associated with higher disease activity, severity and greater mortality in RA [102]. EAM include rheumatoid nodules, ocular inflammation, rheumatoid vasculitis, polyneuropathy, and secondary Sjögren's syndrome [99, 100].

There have been several reports on the relationship between smoking and RA-EAM [99–101, 103, 104]. Turesson et al. reported that smoking at RA diagnosis was one of the main predictors of severe EAM [100]. Kim et al. in multivariate logistic regression analysis demonstrated that the development of EAM was associated with smoking, positive ACPA, and disease duration [101]. Patients with RA who developed severe EAM were more often current smokers in another study group [103]. In the established RA, current cigarette smoking is related to the development of rheumatoid nodules [88, 89, 99, 105, 106].

Cigarette smoking is known to have definite link to the pathogenesis of many vascular diseases, which may support the possibility of a strong causal connection to rheumatoid vasculitis [107]. Smoking was more common in patients with vasculitis [108]. The strength of this association was reinforced by the observation of the downward tendency in rheumatoid vasculitis incidence combined with decreased tobacco smoking over the same period [107].

## Serology (Autoantibodies) Parameters

### *Smoking Status*

The fact that smoking-associated RA risk is limited to the seropositive RA population implicates a role for smoking in the generation of RA-associated autoantibodies [14, 109]. Citrullination is the conversion of the amino acid, arginine into the amino acid, citrulline, which is a post-translational modification [110]. Autoantibodies against citrullinated proteins are specific for RA and found in high levels in the disease [64, 65, 110]. In addition, the citrullination induced by smoking might be the first step in the pathogenic chain of RA [111]. SEs are considered the primary risk factor for increased ACPA production in RA [112]. Carrying one or two SE alleles observed to be a high risk for the development of ACPA-positive RA [113]. In HLA-DR-SE positive RA patients, smoking is known to increase risk of developing ACPA [18, 114]. Krol et al. study [97] demonstrated the interaction between smoking and SE leading to production of ACPA and RF in newly diagnosed treatment-naïve RA patients with active disease.

ACPA concentrations were higher among both current and former smokers compared with never smokers among long standing RA patients [52]. Current smokers had higher RF titer than former smokers and never smokers [87]. Smoking demonstrates a significant relationship between the development of both RF and ACPA in RA cohorts from UK [115]. Moreover, smoking was associated with ACPA positively only in RF positive RA patients, and especially in patient who were strongly RF positive. In the logistic regression model, smoking was independent risk factor for ACPA positivity in RA [115]. Furthermore, disease-specific autoantibodies, including ACPA and RF, were shown to appear several years before the diagnosis of the diseases [116]. In a large study including Japanese volunteers, smoking showed a significant association with high levels of ACPA, while smoking and SE do not have comparable effect in the general population on the production of ACPA and RF as with patients with RA [117].

In a cohort of ACPA-positive RA patients, smoking increases the levels of certain ACPA subclasses, such as Immunoglobulin (Ig) A and IgM, than in non-smokers RA [118]. In the study by Martinsson et al. [119], they described the association of smoking habits across different IgG ACPA subclasses. IgG2 and IgA ACPA were predominantly associated with smoking, while IgG1 and IgG4 related more distinctly to the carriage of SE genes. Roos et al. [120] found that unlike IgG ACPA, circulating serum IgA ACPA, which is present in patients with recent-onset RA, is environmentally linked to cigarette smoking. In this study [120], serum IgA ACPA was associated significantly with smoking (79% ever smokers among IgA ACPA-positive patients vs. 59% in IgA ACPA-negative patients).

***Smoking Intensity***

In the study of Murphy et al. [115], there was a clear relationship between pack/years smoking with RF, and ACPA positivity in RA. Tobacco exposure and heavy smoker (> 20 packs/year) were associated with the presence of ACPA antibodies in patients with RA [42]. For RF, the association was also significant for tobacco exposure and smoking dose among the same RA population. A lower smoking cessation (median years) was observed in ACPA-positive RA cases than in controls, however the intensity of smoking (packs/year) were relatively similar between the cases and the controls who were smokers [24]. However, researchers [115] did not find a relationship between smoking intensity and positivity for ACPA alone, which open a window for the debate that the main determinants of ACPA positivity are RF rather than smoking per se.

***Radiographic Damage***

RA severity is defined by the degree of structural damage and functional disabilities. The effect of smoking on the radiographic progression of RA is not well established and remains controversial. Cigarette smoking was associated increased joint destruction and decreased functional abilities [121–123]. The presence of seropositive (RF, ACPA), is known to be associated with significant radiological progression [124].

Similar associations of smoking status were observed with disease severity measured by multidimensional health assessment questionnaire (MD-HAQ) and pain [52]. The prevalence of joint erosion was particularly higher in seropositive RA patients and in those with a history of smoking only irrespective of SE, which may indicate that smoking enhances the development of erosive disease in RA through distinctive pathways [97]. A previous study showed that smoking was a strong independent risk factor for radiographic progression in early RA [105]. Baseline current smoking along with older age, higher BMI, DAS28 were positive predictors of worse pain at 1 year follow up in RA cohort assembled from the British Society for Rheumatology Biologics Register (BSRBR) [125]. In patients with RA, the erosion narrowing score was higher in current smokers and former smokers than in never smokers. Furthermore, tobacco exposure remained independently associated with simple erosion narrowing score [87]. Furthermore, studies on tobacco smokeless stated no association between usage of snuff and increased disease severity [29, 30].

Even though from the above findings, effect of smoking on RA radiographic erosions score remains debatable [126]. The proportion of erosive disease, radiographic progression and Sharp scores were similar in all smoking categories in RA patients [86, 90]. RA meta-analysis demonstrated that the effect of smoking on joint damage was mediated via ACPA, and smoking was not an independent risk factor for radiological progression [126]. Furthermore, Vesperini et al. described that smoking had no significant effect on RA disease activity and disability. The study in patients with early arthritis showed that smoking reduces radiographic disease progression and speculated that the anti-inflammatory effect of nicotine might explain the lower structural disease progression in RA current smokers [127].

These controversies in the effect of smoking on disease activity and severity may be related to several factors, such as different quantification of smoking, a measurement period, gender or the presence of autoantibodies. Thus, further prospective studies among RA populations are crucial to elucidate the relationship between disease activity and severity with different kind of smoking exposure after controlling of other independent factors.

### *Therapeutic Response*

Smoking status has an influence on RA patients' response to disease modifying anti-rheumatic drugs (DMARDs) [95, 128–130]. Different studies found that RA smokers show a lower response to infliximab, an anti TNF-α therapy [95, 128] and also the poor response to infliximab is linked to the smoking history (pack-year) of patients at the initiation of drug [129]. In a multivariate analysis, smokers under anti TNF-α therapy have a reduced chance of achieving a moderate response on the European League Against Rheumatism (EULAR) response criteria compared to non-smokers [130]. Logistic regression analysis of the RA registry cohorts revealed that current smoking was one of the independent predictors of discontinuation of the first TNF-α inhibitors within 1 year from their initiation, as were female gender, comorbidities, extra-articular manifestations and worse function [125]. The necessity of TNF-α antagonist discontinuation was predicted by current smoking and by the number of previously used biological DMARDs [131]. Using these two predictors, the investigators developed a simple score predicting discontinuation with high positive predictive value.

Westhoff et al. proposed that smoking diminishes the potency of anti-rheumatic drugs [126]. In their prospective study of early RA cohort, current smokers had taken significantly more DMARD combinations or biologics drugs, which may indicate that smoking weakens the potency of these drugs or higher disease activity among smokers that can be controlled by high doses of drugs [126]. Therefore, RA patients who smoke may need a higher dose of DMARDs. The specific mechanism of how smoking decreases the response to anti-rheumatic therapy in RA remains unresolved; however, there are many suggested theories. One possible mechanism to explain the effect of smoking on the response to DMARDs, is the association of high level of antibodies, RF and ACPA with smoking, and in turn these antibodies known to be associated with poor response to anti-TNF-α therapy [132–134]. Others implicate that smoking is associated with high levels of inflammatory cytokines [8, 50, 51], as well as high ratios of TNF-α and serum IL-2 receptor (sIL-2R) than non-smokers [49, 135]. Moreover, Shin et al. suggested that IL-2-sIL-2R system activation reduced the response to TNF-α antagonist in RA patients who smoke [136]. Other factors suggested by Metsios et al., that the metabolism of DMARDs can be higher in RA patients who smoke than non-smokers based on the fact that smoker have accelerated metabolic rate [137]. Stamp et al. showed that smoking could decrease methotrexate polyglutamates levels [138]. In their prospective study of early RA cohort, current smokers had taken significantly more DMARD combinations or biologics drugs, which may indicate that smoking weakens the potency of these drugs or higher disease activity among smokers that can be controlled by high doses of drugs [126]. Therefore, RA patients who smoke may need a higher dose of DMARDs.

## Smoking and RA Comorbidities and Mortality

Cigarette smoking is one of the most important risk factors for development of cardiovascular diseases (CVD) in general; and RA itself is considered as a major risk factor [139]. Tobacco smoking remains the leading cause of preventable death worldwide [140]. In large international cohorts of patients with RA from 13 rheumatology centers conducted on behalf of A Trans-Atlantic Cardiovascular Consortium for RA (ATACC-RA) [141], smoking and hypertension had the highest population attributable risk (PAR) for CVD (myocardial infarction, angina, stroke, peripheral vascular disease and CVD death) overall and among both sexes. PAR for smoking were nearly twice as high among men than women, but these differences did not reach statistical significance.

Kim et al. [142], found that antiphospholipid antibodies (aPL) was present in RA patients who were more often smokers, and was an independent factor for the development of arterial thrombosis. Smoking status (current, previous, never) were significantly different between RA groups divided by presence or absence of aPL, but smoking dose (pack-year) did not differ between the two groups. In the multivariate adjusted model of the same study, only smoking was more likely to increase the risk for the development of aPL, but statistical significance was not attained. These results emphasized that smoking exposure might trigger the development of aPL with subsequent acceleration of CVD in RA patients [142]. This is consistent with the hypothesis that smoking among other environmental factors plays a role in the induction of antiphospholipid syndrome in some people [143].

Joseph et al. [144], found that patients with RA who currently smoke have an increased risk of hospitalizations for cardiovascular events (CVE) and respiratory tract infections (RTI) compared with never and former smokers. The risks of hospitalization for CVE or RTI were more than twice higher in current vs never smokers. In addition, the risks for both outcomes were significantly higher in current compared with former smokers. Women with RA had higher mortality rate than comparators based on the smoking intensity [145]. Smoking >5 pack-years after RA diagnosis significantly increased mortality beyond the risk of non-RA comparators. The mortality burden from smoking for RA patients is higher than the effect observed in the general population [145].

Cigarette smoking was associated with higher lung shrinkage; more pronounced in RA patients than in the general population. These data from a population-based cohort suggest that cigarette smoking may be a potent interstitial lung disease (ILD) risk factor for RA patients than in the general population [146]. In retrospective analysis of 550 patients with RA-associated ILD, Zhang et al. [147] showed that smoking history and positive RF, along with other factors, were closely related to RA-ILD in the final regression model.

Depression was significantly associated with current smoking in subsample of diagnosed RA (extracted from US population based database) [148]. However, in the logistic regression analysis after adjusting for independents, depression lost the association with current smoking [148].

These negative health effects associated with smoking in patients with RA make a convincing way for smoking cessation. Therefore, the advice for the patients to quit smoking is to improve their health and life expectancy, beside the possible effects of smoking on disease activity.

## SMOKING CESSATION IN RA

Given that smoking habit is the most significant modifiable risk for RA, and associated with increased RA disease activity, the detrimental effects of smoking could be reduced through smoking cessation counseling [52], especially in some cases of RA without other risk [40]. Recent study showed that smoking cessation interventions at RA diagnosis may significantly decrease the mortality burden of RA [145]. Moreover, persistent smoking cessation within four years of RA diagnosis reduced mortality risk, with a similar effect observed among non-RA comparators in women among the Nurses' Health Study [145]. Compared to continued smoking, sustained cessation was associated with similarly decreased mortality in both the RA and comparison cohorts [145]. From the same NHS database, women followed prospectively for 26 years, risk of RA for past smokers was similar to the RA risk of non-smoker which persisted for ≥20 years after smoking cessation [19]. Similarly, in the prospective Swedish cohort, risk of RA was still significantly elevated 15 years after smoking cessation compared to never smokers, instead the risk steadily decreased over increasing duration of smoking cessation [149]. In a retrospective study by Joseph et al. [144], for each year of smoking cessation, the risk of first CVE and RTI hospitalization fell significantly, approximately 25% and 15% respectively. These results could be used to help encourage patients with RA to stop smoking.

Recently, tailoring smoking cessation interventions for special populations, such as RA, of smokers has been suggested [150]. Aimer et al., designed a smoking cessation intervention specific for RA patients [151], based on their previous qualitative research identified the RA-related barriers to stop smoking [152]. When this RA-specific smoking cessation intervention had been applied with current RA smokers, it provided useful perception from the participants. However, successful smoking cessation was found to be patient driven and the participants were found to be personally responsible for their own quitting [153]. Later on, based on their subsequent pilot study, Aimer et al. [154], suggested that brief advice and nicotine replacement therapy are currently the best practice for supporting people with RA who wish to quit smoking.

Whether the intensive smoking cessation intervention helps smokers with RA to achieve continuous smoking cessation and whether, it will reduce their RA disease activity is under evaluation in the ongoing open label randomized controlled trial (RCT) [155]. The intervention arm in this multicenter RCT will receive motivational counselling combined with tailored nicotine replacement therapy versus standard care on smoking cessation in the control group. The trial [155] aims to generate high quality evidence for the feasibility of a health promotion intervention for smokers with RA.

## CONCLUSION

This chapter summarized the possible link between smoking and genetics in the susceptibility to RA. The immunological changes that cause RA in smokers have been proposed by several mechanisms, which especially affect genetically predisposed individuals. Additional studies are necessary to evaluate other pathophysiologic associations between smoking exposure and RA risk. Continued exploration of how cigarette smoking affects RA disease status (activity, severity, response to therapy and associated comorbidities) is necessary. Recent studies provide evidence that smoking is associated with accelerated cardiovascular disease, in addition to its influence on the disease and response to anti-rheumatic drugs making it essential to inform RA patients regarding these hazardous effects. Understanding the relationship between smoking and RA may provide the first step in the prevention strategies in high risk individuals. Finally, RA tailored specific smoking cessation programs are emerging.

## References


[1] Symmons DPM. Epidemiology of rheumatoid arthritis: determinants of onset, persistence and outcome. *Best Pract Res Clin Rheumatol.* 2002;16(5):707–22.

[2] Arnett FC, Edworthy SM, Bloch DA, McShane DJ, Fries JF, Cooper NS, et al. The American Rheumatism Association 1987 revised criteria for the classification of rheumatoid arthritis. *Arthritis Rheum.* 1988 Mar;31(3):315–24.

[3] Aletaha D, Neogi T, Silman AJ, Funovits J, Felson DT, Bingham CO, et al. 2010 rheumatoid arthritis classification criteria: an American College of Rheumatology/European League Against Rheumatism collaborative initiative. *Arthritis Rheum.* 2010;62(9):2569–81.

[4] Klareskog L, Malmstrom V, Lundberg K, Padyukov L, Alfredsson L. Smoking, citrullination and genetic variability in the immunopathogenesis of rheumatoid arthritis. *Semin Immunol.* 2011 Apr;23(2):92–8.

[5] Bowes J, Barton A. Recent advances in the genetics of RA susceptibility. *Rheumatology* (Oxford). 2008 Apr;47(4):399–402.

[6] Gregersen PK. Pathways to gene identification in rheumatoid arthritis: PTPN22 and beyond. *Immunol Rev.* 2005 Apr;204:74–86.

[7] MacGregor AJ, Snieder H, Rigby AS, Koskenvuo M, Kaprio J, Aho K, et al. Characterizing the quantitative genetic contribution to rheumatoid arthritis using data from twins. *Arthritis Rheum.* 2000 Jan;43(1):30–7.

[8] Arnson Y, Shoenfeld Y, Amital H. Effects of tobacco smoke on immunity, inflammation and autoimmunity. *J Autoimmun.* 2010 May;34(3):J258-65.

[9] Pryor WA, Stone K, Zang LY, Bermudez E. Fractionation of aqueous cigarette tar extracts: fractions that contain the tar radical cause DNA damage. *Chem Res Toxicol.* 1998 May;11(5):441–8.

[10] Vessey MP, Villard-Mackintosh L, Yeates D. Oral contraceptives, cigarette smoking and other factors in relation to arthritis. *Contraception.* 1987 May;35(5):457–64.

[11] Stolt P, Bengtsson C, Nordmark B, Lindblad S, Lundberg I, Klareskog L, et al. Quantification of the influence of cigarette smoking on rheumatoid arthritis: results from a population based case-control study, using incident cases. *Ann Rheum Dis.* 2003;62(9):835–41.

[12] Di Giuseppe D, Discacciati A, Orsini N, Wolk A. Cigarette smoking and risk of rheumatoid arthritis: a dose-response meta-analysis. *Arthritis Res Ther.* 2014;16(2):R61.

[13] Sugiyama D, Nishimura K, Tamaki K, Tsuji G, Nakazawa T, Morinobu A, et al. Impact of smoking as a risk factor for developing rheumatoid arthritis: a meta-analysis of observational studies. *Ann Rheum Dis.* 2010;69(1):70–81.

[14] Padyukov L, Silva C, Stolt P, Alfredsson L, Klareskog L. A gene-environment interaction between smoking and shared epitope genes in HLA-DR provides a high risk of seropositive rheumatoid arthritis. *Arthritis Rheum.* 2004 Oct;50(10):3085–92.

[15] Heliovaara M, Aho K, Aromaa A, Knekt P, Reunanen A. Smoking and risk of rheumatoid arthritis. *J Rheumatol.* 1993 Nov;20(11):1830–5.

[16] Uhlig T, Hagen KB, Kvien TK. Current tobacco smoking, formal education, and the risk of rheumatoid arthritis. *J Rheumatol.* 1999 Jan;26(1):47–54.

[17] Kallberg H, Ding B, Padyukov L, Bengtsson C, Ronnelid J, Klareskog L, et al. Smoking is a major preventable risk factor for rheumatoid arthritis: estimations of risks after various exposures to cigarette smoke. *Ann Rheum Dis.* 2011 Mar;70(3):508–11.

[18] Klareskog L, Stolt P, Lundberg K, Kallberg H, Bengtsson C, Grunewald J, et al. A new model for an etiology of rheumatoid arthritis: smoking may trigger HLA-DR (shared epitope)-restricted immune reactions to autoantigens modified by citrullination. *Arthritis Rheum.* 2006 Jan;54(1):38–46.

[19] Costenbader KH, Feskanich D, Mandl LA, Karlson EW. Smoking intensity, duration, and cessation, and the risk of rheumatoid arthritis in women. *Am J Med.* 2006 Jun;119(6):503.e1-9.

[20] Fisher BA, Cartwright AJ, Quirke AM, de Pablo P, Romaguera D, Panico S, et al. Smoking, Porphyromonas gingivalis and the immune response to citrullinated autoantigens before the clinical onset of rheumatoid arthritis in a Southern European nested case-control study. *BMC Musculoskelet Disord.* 2015 Nov;16:331.

[21] Jutley G, Raza K, Buckley CD. New pathogenic insights into rheumatoid arthritis. *Curr Opin Rheumatol.* 2015 May;27(3):249–55.

[22] Han B, Diogo D, Eyre S, Kallberg H, Zhernakova A, Bowes J, et al. Fine mapping seronegative and seropositive rheumatoid arthritis to shared and distinct HLA alleles by adjusting for the effects of heterogeneity. *Am J Hum Genet*. 2014 Apr;94(4):522–32.

[23] Xu B, Lin J. Characteristics and risk factors of rheumatoid arthritis in the United States: an NHANES analysis. *PeerJ.* 2017;5:e4035.

[24] Zeng P, Chen Z, Klareskog L, Alfredsson L, Bengtsson C, Jiang X. Amount of smoking, duration of smoking cessation and their interaction with silica exposure in the risk of rheumatoid arthritis among males: results from the Swedish Epidemiological Investigation of Rheumatoid Arthritis (EIRA) study. *Annals of the rheumatic diseases.* England; 2017.

[25] Yin J, He D, Jiang L, Cheng F, Guo Q, Huang S, et al. Influence of Cigarette Smoking on Rheumatoid Arthritis Risk in the Han Chinese Population. Vol. 4, *Frontiers in Medicine.* 2017.

[26] Sparks JA, Chang SC, Deane KD, Gan RW, Kristen Demoruelle M, Feser ML, et al. Associations of Smoking and Age With Inflammatory Joint Signs Among Unaffected First-Degree Relatives of Rheumatoid Arthritis Patients: Results From Studies of the Etiology of Rheumatoid Arthritis. *Arthritis Rheumatol* (Hoboken, NJ). 2016 Aug;68(8):1828–38.

[27] Gritz ER, Baer-Weiss V, Benowitz NL, Van Vunakis H, Jarvik ME. Plasma nicotine and cotinine concentrations in habitual smokeless tobacco users. *Clin Pharmacol Ther. 1*981 Aug;30(2):201–9.

[28] Vincent AO, Steven OA, Felix E, Ize-Iyamu OK, Veronica AA, Jato OE, et al. A comparative evaluation and toxicity assessment of heavy metals in commonly smoked cigarette brands and local tobacco snuff purchased and consumed in Nigeria. *Res J Environ Toxicol.* 2011;5(6):359.

[29] Jiang X, Alfredsson L, Klareskog L, Bengtsson C. Smokeless tobacco (moist snuff) use and the risk of developing rheumatoid arthritis: results from a case-control study. *Arthritis Care Res* (Hoboken). 2014 Oct;66(10):1582–6.

[30] Andersson MLE, Bergman S, Soderlin MK. The effect of snuff (smokeless tobacco) on disease activity and function in rheumatoid arthritis: experiences from the Better Anti-Rheumatic FarmacOTherapy, a longitudinal multicenter study on early rheumatoid arthritis. *J Clin Rheumatol.* 2013 Jan;19(1):14–8.

[31] Karlson EW, Lee IM, Cook NR, Manson JE, Buring JE, Hennekens CH. A retrospective cohort study of cigarette smoking and risk of rheumatoid arthritis in female health professionals. *Arthritis Rheum.* 1999 May;42(5):910–7.

[32] Krishnan E, Sokka T, Hannonen P. Smoking-gender interaction and risk for rheumatoid arthritis. *Arthritis Res Ther.* 2003;5(3):R158-62.

[33] Bang SY, Lee KH, Cho SK, Lee HS, Lee KW, Bae SC. Smoking increases rheumatoid arthritis susceptibility in individuals carrying the HLA-DRB1 shared epitope, regardless of rheumatoid factor or anti-cyclic citrullinated peptide antibody status. *Arthritis Rheum.* 2010 Feb;62(2):369–77.

[34] Taylor LH, Twigg S, Worthington J, Emery P, Morgan AW, Wilson AG, et al. Metaanalysis of the association of smoking and PTPN22 R620W genotype on autoantibody status and radiological erosions in rheumatoid arthritis. *J Rheumatol*. 2013 Jul;40(7):1048–53.

[35] Kallberg H, Padyukov L, Plenge RM, Ronnelid J, Gregersen PK, van der Helm-van Mil AHM, et al. Gene-gene and gene-environment interactions involving HLA-DRB1, PTPN22, and smoking in two subsets of rheumatoid arthritis. *Am J Hum Genet.* 2007 May;80(5):867–75.

[36] Paul BJ, Kandy HI, Krishnan V. Pre-rheumatoid arthritis and its prevention. *Eur J Rheumatol*. 2017 Jun;4(2):161–5.

[37] Freedman AN, Michalek AM, Marshall JR, Mettlin CJ, Petrelli NJ, Zhang ZF, et al. The relationship between smoking exposure and p53 overexpression in colorectal cancer. *Br J Cancer.* 1996 Apr;73(8):902–8.

[38] Reme T, Travaglio A, Gueydon E, Adla L, Jorgensen C, Sany J. Mutations of the p53 tumour suppressor gene in erosive rheumatoid synovial tissue. *Clin Exp Immunol.* 1998 Feb;111(2):353–8.

[39] Firestein GS, Echeverri F, Yeo M, Zvaifler NJ, Green DR. Somatic mutations in the p53 tumor suppressor gene in rheumatoid arthritis synovium. *Proc Natl Acad Sci U S A*. 1997 Sep;94(20):10895–900.

[40] Margulies L, Sehgal PB. Modulation of the human interleukin-6 promoter (IL-6) and transcription factor C/EBP beta (NF-IL6) activity by p53 species. *J Biol Chem.* 1993 Jul;268(20):15096–100.

[41] Silman AJ, Newman J, MacGregor AJ. Cigarette smoking increases the risk of rheumatoid arthritis. Results from a nationwide study of disease-discordant twins. *Arthritis Rheum.* 1996 May;39(5):732–5.

[42] Garcia de Veas Silva JL, Gonzalez Rodriguez C, Hernandez Cruz B. Association of the Shared Epitope, Smoking and the Interaction Between the Two With the Presence of Autoantibodies (Anti-CCP and FR) in Patients With Rheumatoid Arthritis in a Hospital in Seville, Spain. *Reumatol Clin.* 2017 Nov.

[43] Karlson EW, Chang SC, Cui J, Chibnik LB, Fraser PA, De Vivo I, et al. Gene-environment interaction between HLA-DRB1 shared epitope and heavy cigarette smoking in predicting incident rheumatoid arthritis. *Ann Rheum Dis*. 2010 Jan;69(1):54–60.

[44] Sopori M. Effects of cigarette smoke on the immune system. Vol. 2, Nature reviews. *Immunology*. England; 2002. p. 372–7.

[45] Reynolds HY. Bronchoalveolar lavage. *Am Rev Respir Dis*. 1987 Jan;135(1):250–63.

[46] Geusens P. The role of RANK ligand/osteoprotegerin in rheumatoid arthritis. *Ther Adv Musculoskelet Dis*. 2012 Aug;4(4):225–33.

[47] Johannsen A, Susin C, Gustafsson A. Smoking and inflammation: evidence for a synergistic role in chronic disease. *Periodontol* 2000. 2014 Feb;64(1):111–26.

[48] Bermudez EA, Rifai N, Buring JE, Manson JE, Ridker PM. Relation between markers of systemic vascular inflammation and smoking in women. *Am J Cardiol.* 2002 May;89(9):1117–9.

[49] Glossop JR, Dawes PT, Mattey DL. Association between cigarette smoking and release of tumour necrosis factor alpha and its soluble receptors by peripheral blood mononuclear cells in patients with rheumatoid arthritis. *Rheumatology* (Oxford). 2006 Oct;45(10):1223–9.

[50] Harel-Meir M, Sherer Y, Shoenfeld Y. Tobacco smoking and autoimmune rheumatic diseases. *Nat Clin Pract Rheumatol.* 2007;3(12):707–15.

[51] Yoshida Y, Tanaka T. Interleukin 6 and rheumatoid arthritis. *Biomed Res Int.* 2014;2014:698313.

[52] Sokolove J, Wagner CA, Lahey LJ, Sayles H, Duryee MJ, Reimold AM, et al. Increased inflammation and disease activity among current cigarette smokers with rheumatoid arthritis: a cross-sectional analysis of US veterans. *Rheumatology* (Oxford). 2016 Nov;55(11):1969–77.

[53] Harrison OJ, Foley J, Bolognese BJ, Long E 3rd, Podolin PL, Walsh PT. Airway infiltration of CD4+ CCR6+ Th17 type cells associated with chronic cigarette smoke induced airspace enlargement. *Immunol Lett*. 2008 Nov;121(1):13–21.

[54] Benedetti G, Miossec P. Interleukin 17 contributes to the chronicity of inflammatory diseases such as rheumatoid arthritis. *Eur J Immunol.* 2014 Feb;44(2):339–47.

[55] Lacey DL, Timms E, Tan HL, Kelley MJ, Dunstan CR, Burgess T, et al. Osteoprotegerin ligand is a cytokine that regulates osteoclast differentiation and activation. *Cell.* 1998 Apr;93(2):165–76.

[56] Lappin DF, Sherrabeh S, Jenkins WMM, Macpherson LMD. Effect of smoking on serum RANKL and OPG in sex, age and clinically matched supportive-therapy periodontitis patients. *J Clin Periodontol.* 2007 Apr;34(4):271–7.

[57] Bracke K, Cataldo D, Maes T, Gueders M, Noel A, Foidart JM, et al. Matrix metalloproteinase-12 and cathepsin D expression in pulmonary macrophages and dendritic cells of cigarette smoke-exposed mice. *Int Arch Allergy Immunol.* 2005 Oct;138(2):169–79.

[58] Liu Y, Aryee MJ, Padyukov L, Fallin MD, Hesselberg E, Runarsson A, et al. Epigenome-wide association data implicate DNA methylation as an intermediary of genetic risk in rheumatoid arthritis. *Nat Biotechnol.* 2013 Feb;31(2):142–7.

[59] Xue M, McKelvey K, Shen K, Minhas N, March L, Park SY, et al. Endogenous MMP-9 and not MMP-2 promotes rheumatoid synovial fibroblast survival, inflammation and cartilage degradation. *Rheumatology* (Oxford). 2014 Dec;53(12):2270–9.

[60] Raitio A, Tuomas H, Kokkonen N, Salo T, Sorsa T, Hanemaaijer R, et al. Levels of matrix metalloproteinase-2, -9 and -8 in the skin, serum and saliva of smokers and non-smokers. *Arch Dermatol Res.* 2005 Dec;297(6):242–8.

[61] Yanbaeva DG, Dentener MA, Creutzberg EC, Wesseling G, Wouters EFM. Systemic effects of smoking. *Chest.* 2007 May;131(5):1557–66.

[62] Ruiz-Esquide V, Sanmarti R. Tobacco and other environmental risk factors in rheumatoid arthritis. *Reumatol Clin.* 2012;8(6):342–50.

[63] Hoovestol RA, Mikuls TR. Environmental exposures and rheumatoid arthritis risk. *Curr Rheumatol Rep.* 2011 Oct;13(5):431–9.

[64] Scott DL, Wolfe F, Huizinga TWJ. Rheumatoid arthritis. *Lancet* (London, England). 2010 Sep;376(9746):1094–108.

[65] Cooles FAH, Isaacs JD. Pathophysiology of rheumatoid arthritis. *Curr Opin Rheumatol.* 2011 May;23(3):233–40.

[66] Pryor WA, Stone K. Oxidants in cigarette smoke. Radicals, hydrogen peroxide, peroxynitrate, and peroxynitrite. *Ann N Y Acad Sci*. 1993 May;686:12–8.

[67] Kalpakcioglu B, Senel K. The interrelation of glutathione reductase, catalase, glutathione peroxidase, superoxide dismutase, and glucose-6-phosphate in the pathogenesis of rheumatoid arthritis. *Clin Rheumatol.* 2008 Feb;27(2):141–5.

[68] Hagiwara E, Takahashi KI, Okubo T, Ohno S, Ueda A, Aoki A, et al. Cigarette smoking depletes cells spontaneously secreting th1cytokines in the human airway. *Cytokine.* 2001;14(2):121–6.

[69] Lindblad SS, Mydel P, Jonsson M, Senior RM, Tarkowski A, Bokarewa M. Smoking and nicotine exposure delay development of collagen-induced arthritis in mice. *Arthritis Res Ther.* 2009;11(3):R88.

[70] Kalayciyan A, Orawa H, Fimmel S, Perschel FH, Gonzalez JB, Fitzner RG, et al. Nicotine and biochanin A, but not cigarette smoke, induce anti-inflammatory effects on keratinocytes and endothelial cells in patients with Behcet's disease. *J Invest Dermatol.* 2007 Jan;127(1):81–9.

[71] Yu H, Yang YH, Rajaiah R, Moudgil KD. Nicotine-induced differential modulation of autoimmune arthritis in the Lewis rat involves changes in interleukin-17 and anti-cyclic citrullinated peptide antibodies. *Arthritis Rheum.* 2011 Apr;63(4):981–91.

[72] Johnson JD, Houchens DP, Kluwe WM, Craig DK, Fisher GL. Effects of mainstream and environmental tobacco smoke on the immune system in animals and humans: a review. *Crit Rev Toxicol.* 1990;20(5):369–95.

[73] Dale DC, Boxer L, Liles WC. The phagocytes: neutrophils and monocytes. *Blood.* 2008 Aug;112(4):935–45.

[74] Corberand J, Nguyen F, Do AH, Dutau G, Laharrague P, Fontanilles AM, et al. Effect of tobacco smoking on the functions of polymorphonuclear leukocytes. *Infect Immun.* 1979;23(3):577–81.

[75] Shegarfi H, Naddafi F, Mirshafiey A. Natural killer cells and their role in rheumatoid arthritis: friend or foe? *Scientific World Journal.* 2012;2012:491974.

[76] Wasen C, Turkkila M, Bossios A, Erlandsson M, Andersson KM, Ekerljung L, et al. Smoking activates cytotoxic CD8(+) T cells and causes survivin release in rheumatoid arthritis. *J Autoimmun.* 2017 Mar;78:101–10.

[77] Huber LC, Distler O, Tarner I, Gay RE, Gay S, Pap T. Synovial fibroblasts: key players in rheumatoid arthritis. *Rheumatology* (Oxford). 2006 Jun;45(6):669–75.

[78] Bartok B, Firestein GS. Fibroblast-like synoviocytes: key effector cells in rheumatoid arthritis. *Immunol Rev.* 2010 Jan;233(1):233–55.

[79] Shizu M, Itoh Y, Sunahara R, Chujo S, Hayashi H, Ide Y, et al. Cigarette smoke condensate upregulates the gene and protein expression of proinflammatory cytokines in human fibroblast-like synoviocyte line. *J Interferon Cytokine Res.* 2008 Aug;28(8):509–21.

[80] Santoro MG. Heat shock factors and the control of the stress response. *Biochem Pharmacol.* 2000 Jan;59(1):55–63.

[81] Bijl M, Horst G, Limburg PC, Kallenberg CG. Effects of smoking on activation markers, Fas expression and apoptosis of peripheral blood lymphocytes. *Eur J Clin Invest.* 2001 Jun;31(6):550–3.

[82] Cheng XL, Zhang H, Guo D, Qiao ZD. Upregulation of Fas and FasL expression in nicotine-induced apoptosis of endothelial cells. *Methods Find Exp Clin Pharmacol.* 2010;32(1):13–8.

[83] Imirzalioglu P, Uckan S, Alaaddinoglu EE, Haberal A, Uckan D. Cigarette smoking and apoptosis. *J Periodontol.* 2005 May;76(5):737–9.

[84] Zeilinger S, Kuhnel B, Klopp N, Baurecht H, Kleinschmidt A, Gieger C, et al. Tobacco smoking leads to extensive genome-wide changes in DNA methylation. *PLoS One.* 2013;8(5):e63812.

[85] Viatte S, Plant D, Raychaudhuri S. Genetics and epigenetics of rheumatoid arthritis. *Nat Rev Rheumatol.* 2013 Mar;9(3):141–53.

[86] Manfredsdottir VF, Vikingsdottir T, Jonsson T, Geirsson AJ, Kjartansson O, Heimisdottir M, et al. The effects of tobacco smoking and rheumatoid factor seropositivity on disease activity and joint damage in early rheumatoid arthritis. *Rheumatology.* 2006;45(6):734–40.

[87] Haye Salinas MJ, Retamozo S, Alvarez AC, Maldonado Ficco H, Dal Pra F, Citera G, et al. Effects of cigarette smoking on early arthritis: a cross-sectional study-data from the Argentine Consortium for Early Arthritis (CONAART). *Rheumatol Int.* 2015 May;35(5):855–9.

[88] Saevarsdottir S, Wedren S, Seddighzadeh M, Bengtsson C, Wesley A, Lindblad S, et al. Patients with early rheumatoid arthritis who smoke are less likely to respond to treatment with methotrexate and tumor necrosis factor inhibitors: observations from the Epidemiological Investigation of Rheumatoid Arthritis and the Swedish Rheumatology Re. *Arthritis Rheum.* 2011 Jan;63(1):26–36.

[89] Sokka T, Hetland ML, Makinen H, Kautiainen H, Horslev-Petersen K, Luukkainen RK, et al. Remission and rheumatoid arthritis: data on patients receiving usual care in twenty-four countries. *Arthritis Rheum.* 2008 Sep;58(9):2642–51.

[90] Quintana-Duque MA, Rondon-Herrera F, Calvo-Paramo E, Yunis JJ, Varela-Narino A, Iglesias-Gamarra A. The impact of smoking on disease activity, disability, and radiographic damage in rheumatoid arthritis: is cigarette protective? *Rheumatol Int.* 2017 Dec;37(12):2065–70.

[91] Papadopoulos NG, Alamanos Y, Voulgari P V, Epagelis EK, Tsifetaki N, Drosos AA. Does cigarette smoking influence disease expression, activity and severity in early rheumatoid arthritis patients? *Clin Exp Rheumatol.* 2005;23(6):861.

[92] Rojas-Serrano J, Perez LL, Garcia CG, Moctezuma F, Alvarez-Hernandez E, Vazquez-Mellado J, et al. Current smoking status is associated to a non-ACR 50 response in early rheumatoid arthritis. A cohort study. *Clin Rheumatol.* 2011 Dec;30(12):1589–93.

[93] Forslind K, Hafstrom I, Ahlmen M, Svensson B. Sex: a major predictor of remission in early rheumatoid arthritis? *Ann Rheum Dis*. 2007 Jan;66(1):46–52.

[94] Inoue Y, Nakajima A, Tanaka E, Inoue E, Kobayashi A, Hoshi D, et al. Effect of Smoking on Remission Proportions Differs Between Male and Female Patients with Rheumatoid Arthritis: A Study Based on the IORRA Survey. *J Rheumatol.* 2015 Jul;42(7):1083–9.

[95] Hyrich KL, Watson KD, Silman AJ, Symmons DPM. Predictors of response to anti-TNF-alpha therapy among patients with rheumatoid arthritis: results from the British Society for Rheumatology Biologics Register. *Rheumatology* (Oxford). 2006 Dec;45(12):1558–65.

[96] Naranjo A, Toloza S, Guimaraes da Silveira I, Lazovskis J, Hetland ML, Hamoud H, et al. Smokers and non smokers with rheumatoid arthritis have similar clinical status: data from the multinational QUEST-RA database. *Clin Exp Rheumatol.* 2010;28(6):820–7.

[97] Krol A, Garred P, Heegaard NHH, Christensen AF, Hetland ML, Stengaard-Pedersen K, et al. Interactions between smoking, increased serum levels of anti-CCP antibodies, rheumatoid factors, and erosive joint disease in patients with early, untreated rheumatoid arthritis. *Scand J Rheumatol.* 2015;44(1):8–12.

[98] Hammam N, Gheita TA. Impact of secondhand smoking on disease activity in women with rheumatoid arthritis. *Clin Rheumatol.* 2017.

[99] Moura MC, Zakszewski PTS, Silva MBG, Skare TL. Epidemiological profile of patients with extra-articular manifestations of rheumatoid arthritis from the city of Curitiba, south of Brazil. *Rev Bras Reumatol*. 2012 Oct;52(5):679–94.

[100] Turesson C, O'Fallon WM, Crowson CS, Gabriel SE, Matteson EL. Extra-articular disease manifestations in rheumatoid arthritis: incidence trends and risk factors over 46 years. *Ann Rheum Dis.* 2003 Aug;62(8):722–7.

[101] Kim SK, Park SH, Shin IH, Choe JY. Anti-cyclic citrullinated peptide antibody, smoking, alcohol consumption, and disease duration as risk factors for extraarticular manifestations in Korean

patients with rheumatoid arthritis. *J Rheumatol.* 2008 Jun;35(6):995–1001.

[102] Turesson C, Jacobsson LTH. Epidemiology of extra-articular manifestations in rheumatoid arthritis. *Scand J Rheumatol.* 2004;33(2):65–72.

[103] Nyhall-Wahlin BM, Petersson IF, Nilsson JA, Jacobsson LTH, Turesson C. High disease activity disability burden and smoking predict severe extra-articular manifestations in early rheumatoid arthritis. *Rheumatology* (Oxford). 2009 Apr;48(4):416–20.

[104] de Rooy DPC, van Nies JAB, Kapetanovic MC, Kristjansdottir H, Andersson MLE, Forslind K, et al. Smoking as a risk factor for the radiological severity of rheumatoid arthritis: a study on six cohorts. *Ann Rheum Dis.* 2014 Jul;73(7):1384–7.

[105] Nagai S, Hoshino Y, Hayashi M, Ito I. Smoking-related interstitial lung diseases. *Curr Opin Pulm Med.* 2000 Sep;6(5):415–9.

[106] Nyhäll-Wåhlin BM, Jacobsson LTH, Petersson IF, Turesson C. Smoking is a strong risk factor for rheumatoid nodules in early rheumatoid arthritis. *Ann Rheum Dis*. 2006;65(5):601–6.

[107] Albano SA, Santana-Sahagun E, Weisman MH. Cigarette smoking and rheumatoid arthritis. *Semin Arthritis Rheum.* 2001 Dec;31(3):146–59.

[108] Struthers GR, Scott DL, Delamere JP, Sheppeard H, Kitt M. Smoking and rheumatoid vasculitis. *Rheumatol Int.* 1981;1(3):145–6.

[109] Goodson NJ, Farragher TM, Symmons DPM. Rheumatoid factor, smoking, and disease severity: associations with mortality in rheumatoid arthritis. Vol. 35, *The Journal of rheumatology.* Canada; 2008. p. 945–9.

[110] Wegner N, Lundberg K, Kinloch A, Fisher B, Malmstrom V, Feldmann M, et al. Autoimmunity to specific citrullinated proteins gives the first clues to the etiology of rheumatoid arthritis. *Immunol Rev.* 2010 Jan;233(1):34–54.

[111] Reynisdottir G, Karimi R, Joshua V, Olsen H, Hensvold AH, Harju A, et al. Structural changes and antibody enrichment in the lungs are early features of anti-citrullinated protein antibody-positive rheumatoid arthritis. *Arthritis Rheumatol* (Hoboken, NJ). 2014 Jan;66(1):31–9.
[112] Klareskog L, Widhe M, Hermansson M, Ronnelid J. Antibodies to citrullinated proteins in arthritis: pathology and promise. *Curr Opin Rheumatol.* 2008 May;20(3):300–5.
[113] van der Helm-van Mil AHM, Verpoort KN, le Cessie S, Huizinga TWJ, de Vries RRP, Toes REM. The HLA-DRB1 shared epitope alleles differ in the interaction with smoking and predisposition to antibodies to cyclic citrullinated peptide. *Arthritis Rheum.* 2007 Feb;56(2):425–32.
[114] Mattey DL, Dawes PT, Clarke S, Fisher J, Brownfield A, Thomson W, et al. Relationship among the HLA-DRB1 shared epitope, smoking, and rheumatoid factor production in rheumatoid arthritis. *Arthritis Rheum.* 2002 Aug;47(4):403–7.
[115] Murphy D, Mattey D, Hutchinson D. Anti-citrullinated protein antibody positive rheumatoid arthritis is primarily determined by rheumatoid factor titre and the shared epitope rather than smoking per se. *PLoS One.* 2017;12(7):e0180655.
[116] Nielsen SF, Bojesen SE, Schnohr P, Nordestgaard BG. Elevated rheumatoid factor and long term risk of rheumatoid arthritis: a prospective cohort study. *BMJ.* 2012 Sep;345:e5244.
[117] Terao C, Ohmura K, Ikari K, Kawaguchi T, Takahashi M, Setoh K, et al. Effects of smoking and shared epitope on the production of anti-citrullinated peptide antibody in a Japanese adult population. *Arthritis Care Res* (Hoboken). 2014 Dec;66(12):1818–27.
[118] Verpoort KN, Papendrecht-van der Voort EAM, van der Helm-van Mil AHM, Jol-van der Zijde CM, van Tol MJD, Drijfhout JW, et al. Association of smoking with the constitution of the anti-cyclic citrullinated peptide response in the absence of HLA-DRB1 shared epitope alleles. *Arthritis Rheum.* 2007 Sep;56(9):2913–8.

[119] Martinsson K, Johansson A, Kastbom A, Skogh T. Immunoglobulin (Ig)G1 and IgG4 anti-cyclic citrullinated peptide (CCP) associate with shared epitope, whereas IgG2 anti-CCP associates with smoking in patients with recent-onset rheumatoid arthritis (the Swedish TIRA project). *Clin Exp Immunol.* 2017 Apr;188(1):53–62.

[120] Roos K, Martinsson K, Ziegelasch M, Sommarin Y, Svard A, Skogh T, et al. Circulating secretory IgA antibodies against cyclic citrullinated peptides in early rheumatoid arthritis associate with inflammatory activity and smoking. *Arthritis Res Ther.* 2016 May;18(1):119.

[121] Saag KG, Cerhan JR, Kolluri S, Ohashi K, Hunninghake GW, Schwartz DA. Cigarette smoking and rheumatoid arthritis severity. *Ann Rheum Dis.* 1997 Aug;56(8):463–9.

[122] Wolfe F. The effect of smoking on clinical, laboratory, and radiographic status in rheumatoid arthritis. *J Rheumatol.* 2000 Mar;27(3):630–7.

[123] Masdottir B, Jonsson T, Manfredsdottir V, Vikingsson A, Brekkan A, Valdimarsson H. Smoking, rheumatoid factor isotypes and severity of rheumatoid arthritis. *Rheumatology* (Oxford). 2000 Nov;39(11):1202–5.

[124] Klareskog L, Padyukov L, Alfredsson L. Smoking as a trigger for inflammatory rheumatic diseases. *Curr Opin Rheumatol.* 2007;19(1):49–54.

[125] McWilliams DF, Walsh DA. Factors predicting pain and early discontinuation of tumour necrosis factor-alpha-inhibitors in people with rheumatoid arthritis: results from the British society for rheumatology biologics register. *BMC Musculoskelet Disord.* 2016 Aug;17:337.

[126] Westhoff G, Rau R, Zink A. Rheumatoid arthritis patients who smoke have a higher need for DMARDs and feel worse, but they do not have more joint damage than non-smokers of the same serological group. *Rheumatology.* 2008;47(6):849–54.

[127] Vesperini V, Lukas C, Fautrel B, Le Loet X, Rincheval N, Combe B. Association of tobacco exposure and reduction of radiographic progression in early rheumatoid arthritis: results from a French multicenter cohort. *Arthritis Care Res* (Hoboken). 2013 Dec;65(12):1899–906.

[128] Soderlin MK, Petersson IF, Geborek P. The effect of smoking on response and drug survival in rheumatoid arthritis patients treated with their first anti-TNF drug. *Scand J Rheumatol.* 2012 Feb;41(1):1–9.

[129] Mattey DL, Brownfield A, Dawes PT. Relationship between pack-year history of smoking and response to tumor necrosis factor antagonists in patients with rheumatoid arthritis. *J Rheumatol.* 2009 Jun;36(6):1180–7.

[130] Abhishek A, Butt S, Gadsby K, Zhang W, Deighton CM. Anti-TNF-alpha agents are less effective for the treatment of rheumatoid arthritis in current smokers. *J Clin Rheumatol.* 2010 Jan;16(1):15–8.

[131] Cuppen BVJ, Jacobs JWG, Ter Borg EJ, Marijnissen ACA, Bijlsma JWJ, Lafeber FPJG, et al. Necessity of TNF-alpha inhibitor discontinuation in rheumatoid arthritis is predicted by smoking and number of previously used biological DMARDs. *Clin Exp Rheumatol.* 2017;35(2):221–8.

[132] Bobbio-Pallavicini F, Caporali R, Alpini C, Avalle S, Epis OM, Klersy C, et al. High IgA rheumatoid factor levels are associated with poor clinical response to tumour necrosis factor alpha inhibitors in rheumatoid arthritis. *Ann Rheum Dis.* 2007 Mar;66(3):302–7.

[133] Braun-Moscovici Y, Markovits D, Zinder O, Schapira D, Rozin A, Ehrenburg M, et al. Anti-cyclic citrullinated protein antibodies as a predictor of response to anti-tumor necrosis factor-alpha therapy in patients with rheumatoid arthritis. *J Rheumatol.* 2006 Mar;33(3):497–500.

[134] Lee DM, Phillips R, Hagan EM, Chibnik LB, Costenbader KH, Schur PH. Quantifying anti-cyclic citrullinated peptide titres: clinical utility and association with tobacco exposure in patients

with rheumatoid arthritis. *Ann Rheum Dis.* 2009 Feb;68(2):201–8.

[135] Tollerud DJ, Weiss ST, Leung DY. Elevated soluble interleukin-2 receptors in young healthy cigarette smokers: lack of association with atopy or airways hyperresponsiveness. *Int Arch Allergy Immunol.* 1992;97(1):25–30.

[136] Park SJ, Shin JI. The effect of smoking on response and drug survival in rheumatoid arthritis patients treated with their first anti-TNF drug: comments on the article by Soderlin et al. Vol. 41, *Scandinavian journal of rheumatology.* England; 2012. p. 411–2.

[137] Metsios GS, Stavropoulos-Kalinoglou A, Nevill AM, Douglas KMJ, Koutedakis Y, Kitas GD. Cigarette smoking significantly increases basal metabolic rate in patients with rheumatoid arthritis. *Ann Rheum Dis.* 2008;67(1):70–3.

[138] Stamp LK, O'Donnell JL, Chapman PT, Zhang M, Frampton C, James J, et al. Determinants of red blood cell methotrexate polyglutamate concentrations in rheumatoid arthritis patients receiving long-term methotrexate treatment. *Arthritis Rheum.* 2009 Aug;60(8):2248–56.

[139] Crowson CS, Liao KP, Davis JM 3rd, Solomon DH, Matteson EL, Knutson KL, et al. Rheumatoid arthritis and cardiovascular disease. *Am Heart J.* 2013 Oct;166(4):622–628.e1.

[140] Wipfli H. The Tobacco Atlas, Fourth Edition. *Am J Epidemiol* [Internet]. 2012 Dec 15;176(12):1193. Available from: http://dx.doi.org/10.1093/aje/kws389.

[141] Crowson CS, Rollefstad S, Ikdahl E, Kitas GD, van Riel PLCM, Gabriel SE, et al. Impact of risk factors associated with cardiovascular outcomes in patients with rheumatoid arthritis. *Ann Rheum Dis*. 2018 Jan;77(1):48–54.

[142] Kim KJ, Baek IW, Park KS, Kim WU, Cho CS. Association between antiphospholipid antibodies and arterial thrombosis in patients with rheumatoid arthritis. *Lupus.* 2017 Jan;26(1):88–94.

[143] Binder SR, Litwin CM. Anti-phospholipid Antibodies and Smoking: An Overview. *Clin Rev Allergy Immunol.* 2017 Aug;53(1):1–13.

[144] Joseph RM, Movahedi M, Dixon WG, Symmons DP. Risks of smoking and benefits of smoking cessation on hospitalisations for cardiovascular events and respiratory infection in patients with rheumatoid arthritis: a retrospective cohort study using the Clinical Practice Research Datalink. *RMD open.* 2017;3(2):e000506.

[145] Sparks JA, Chang S, Nguyen UDT, Barbhaiya M, Tedeschi SK, Lu B, et al. Smoking behavior changes in the early rheumatoid arthritis period and risk of mortality during 36 years of prospective follow-up. *Arthritis Care Res* (Hoboken). 2017.

[146] Johnson C, Giles JT, Bathon J, Lederer D, Hoffman EA, Barr RG, et al. Smoking and Subclinical ILD in RA versus the Multi-Ethnic Study of Atherosclerosis. *PLoS One.* 2016;11(4):e0153024.

[147] Zhang Y, Li H, Wu N, Dong X, Zheng Y. Retrospective study of the clinical characteristics and risk factors of rheumatoid arthritis-associated interstitial lung disease. *Clin Rheumatol.* 2017 Apr;36(4):817–23.

[148] Xiao Y, Zhao N. Current cigarette use in rheumatoid arthritis patients: associated factors and a limited mediating role of depression. *Rheumatol Int.* 2015 Jul;35(7):1219–24.

[149] Di Giuseppe D, Orsini N, Alfredsson L, Askling J, Wolk A. Cigarette smoking and smoking cessation in relation to risk of rheumatoid arthritis in women. *Arthritis Res Ther.* 2013;15(2):R56.

[150] Borrelli B. Smoking cessation: next steps for special populations research and innovative treatments. Vol. 78, *Journal of consulting and clinical psychology.* United States; 2010. p. 1–12.

[151] Aimer P, Stamp LK, Stebbings S, Cameron V, Kirby S, Croft S, et al. Developing a Tailored Smoking Cessation Intervention for Rheumatoid Arthritis Patients. *Musculoskeletal Care.* 2016 Mar;14(1):2–14.

[152] Aimer P, Stamp L, Stebbings S, Valentino N, Cameron V, Treharne GJ. Identifying barriers to smoking cessation in rheumatoid arthritis. *Arthritis Care Res* (Hoboken). 2015 May;67(5):607–15.

[153] Aimer P, Stamp LK, Stebbings S, Cameron V, Kirby S, Treharne GJ. Exploring perceptions of a rheumatoid arthritis-specific smoking cessation programme. *Musculoskeletal Care.* 2017 Jul.

[154] Aimer P, Treharne GJ, Stebbings S, Frampton C, Cameron V, Kirby S, et al. Efficacy of a Rheumatoid Arthritis-Specific Smoking Cessation Program: A Randomized Controlled Pilot Trial. *Arthritis Care Res* (Hoboken). 2017 Jan;69(1):28–37.

[155] Roelsgaard IK, Thomsen T, Ostergaard M, Christensen R, Hetland ML, Jacobsen S, et al. The effect of an intensive smoking cessation intervention on disease activity in patients with rheumatoid arthritis: study protocol for a randomised controlled trial. *Trials.* 2017 Nov;18(1):570.

# INDEX

## B



## C

## D



## E

## J



## K



## L

## M



## N



## O